Free My Back

Seven Steps to Freedom from Chronic Back Pain

By

Lisa Marie Keller

2014

Dedicated to my parents and grandparents
who helped form me into the person I am today.
I could not have done it without your unwavering
love and support – Thank YOU!!!

I also want to thank my
friends whom I may have alienated while
I was busy working. Thank you for your
understanding and, most of all, your words
of encouragement Jen, Mike and Jeffie.
I love and appreciate all of you.

Free My Back – 7 Steps To Freedom From Chronic Back Pain

Copyright © 2014 Lisa Marie Keller and www.lisamariekeller.com

Published in Wadsworth, Ohio

First edition published 2014, Wadsworth, Ohio

Table of Contents

LEARNING OBJECTIVES AND GOALS..5
CHAPTER 1..6
    You Are Not Alone With Back Pain..6
CHAPTER 2..10
    Understanding My Back..10
CHAPTER 3..16
    Eliminate Back Spasms!...16
CHAPTER 4..23
    Retrain Your Back to Move Right..23
CHAPTER 5..30
    Muscular Support 30
CHAPTER 6..44
    Mental Emotional Pain..44
CHAPTER 7..50
    Help Me Heal 50
Chapter 8..59
    Tools for Trigger Points..59
Chapter 9..63
    Wrapping It Up...63
PICTURE INDEX...65

LEARNING OBJECTIVES AND GOALS

OVERALL LEARNING OUTCOME:

You will follow a seven step system to resolve your chronic back pain without surgery.

SEGMENT LEARNING OBJECTIVES:

1. You will be able to identify and describe the most over-looked and under-treated spot in relation to back pain.

2. You will be able to eliminate your back spasms using a variety of approaches

3. You will be able to implement a very effective technique to retrain your back so it will move the way it originally was designed to move.

4. You will implement the perfect exercises to support your back and develop the right muscle support throughout your healing process.

5. You will identify and eliminate your mental-emotional contributors to your pain.

6. You will be able to determine the best bodyworker to support you in your healing process.

7. You will learn how to use tools to manage your trigger points.

CHAPTER 1

You Are Not Alone With Back Pain

You are experiencing back pain, which means you are one of the majority of Americans today. It is estimated eighty percent of the population will experience back pain at some point in their lives. Back pain is the second most common reason for doctor visits and is surpassed only by upper respiratory infections. It is most definitely an expensive problem as well. I am sure you are fully aware of that given your current experience.

Back pain is the most common reason for missing work. Back pain costs the American public an estimated $50 billion annually. Those are just the costs can be identified with surveys. Back pain affects your lifestyle in ways that cannot be measured, such as slowing you down, causing fatigue, limiting what you can do, disrupting sleep, and making things in life hard to enjoy. The worst part is it makes relaxation nearly impossible. It is safe to say back pain is a serious problem. I am certain you would agree, especially since you are sitting and fidgeting in your chair. I am sure you are trying to find the most comfortable position and get away from the pain. Meanwhile, you are worrying about how you are going to get everything done in your day with pain holding you back.

A large percentage of individuals who have back pain have it for a long time, making it a chronic condition. Spinal fusion surgeries have increased by 220 percent in recent years within the Medicare population alone. Epidural steroid injections among the same population have increased by 629 percent during the same time. Unfortunately, these procedures have not led to an improved quality of life, which is a huge problem. Chronic back pain is a definite part of our lives. It plagues you and numerous others, at great costs to your enjoyment of life. There are also massive financial costs for everyone involved, not just the person with chronic back pain. It is necessary to look at this picture differently. It is necessary to start doing something differently. The definition of insanity is doing the same thing over and over and expecting a different result. Now, let's do something different so we can get a different result.

Are you with me on this? I am right here with you! I have taken numerous people successfully through their chronic back pain, helping them find the light at the end of the tunnel, becoming pain-free without drugs or surgery. I am not a big fan of pharmaceutical drugs (actually I should say my body is not since it reacts badly), and I am terrified of getting any sort of surgery. So those are two options I have not even considered for myself, or as part of my system for resolving chronic pain.

Today, you will be taken through the system I developed for my patients to resolve their chronic back pain. You will be going through a seven-step system, and when you get to the end, you will have a surefire approach for resolving your chronic back pain. This process may have similar steps to other things you have tried, and other steps will be completely foreign to you. That is okay. Remember, you have to do something differently if you want a different result; so keep an open mind through these steps. Okay, so let's go... If you are not on board with trying something different, that is completely okay. I want you to respect your own feelings. However, if that is the case, you may want to stop here since this information may not be a good fit for you :-) Otherwise let's move forward!!!

You may be wondering how to use this book to implement the steps into your life so you can **Free Your Back**. Each step of this system is divided into chapters. Dependent on your learning style, you may want to take it one chapter at a time. This will allow you time to absorb the information within each chapter before moving onto the next. This is how I recommend you go through this book. However, I know what it's like is to be impatient, and to have that desire to get all the information at one time. I am definitely one of those impatient people who wants it all at once; so if you are like me that is totally okay. It is a bit harder that way (trust me, I know from experience), but definitely not impossible. If you are the impatient, want-it-all-at-once type, then I recommend you read through the entire book once, without implementing anything. Then after you have read the entire book, read through it again, taking it one chapter at a time. This will allow you the time to implement each chapter before moving onto the next.

It may take you anywhere from one to seven days to implement each chapter fully before moving onto the next. Take your time and try not to rush the process. Please remember-true healing is a process, and unfortunately, it cannot be rushed. I know it can be discouraging! I fully understand since I wanted my healing to happen yesterday, too. Please be patient with yourself and your body.

You can go through the book in whatever chapter order suits you. Maybe one chapter really interests and excites you, so by all means, start there. Just make sure you go through all of the chapters until the end, making an effort to implement each one. Chapters may seem as though they just are not working for you, or you just are not comfortable with them, and that is okay. It may be worthwhile for you to try those chapters again later after some healing has occurred. You may find you are more receptive at that time. I have found using all parts of this system was most effective in getting lasting and effective healing from back pain for me, and for my patients.

So you have an idea of what to expect, here is a synopsis of the system's steps. First, you are going to gain an understanding of your back. You are going to understand how the sacroiliac joint is one of the most overlooked and under-treated causes of back pain. You will gain an understanding of the pelvic bones that make up the sacroiliac joint, along with the muscles involved.

After gaining a thorough understanding of your back's anatomy, then you will learn how to get rid of your muscle spasms using several approaches. Getting rid of your muscle spasms will help you increase your ability to move and your ability to sleep and relax. Next, you will learn a cutting-edge technique to re-train your back and sacroiliac joint to move the way they originally were designed. It is the foundation of this seven-step system for getting rid of your chronic back pain for good. Re-training your back will allow your body to move more easily and with less effort and, of course, with less pain. Once your back and sacroiliac joints are moving the way they are supposed to, you will need to strengthen the appropriate muscles to support new movement. You will learn that in Chapter 5.

For those of you who understand there is an emotional component to pain, the next chapter will be easy. However, for most people, Chapter 6 may be a new concept. This does not negate its importance! The mental-emotional component of pain can hold you back from healing completely. Because the mental-emotional side can be so instrumental in holding you back from full and efficient healing, it is very important to address this problem. I know from personal experience.

The next chapter is devoted to helping discover what a bodyworker is, and finding out what type of bodyworker is best for you. Through the healing process, you may find having a supportive bodyworker at your side to help you is of utmost importance. It can be difficult to find the right bodyworker. This chapter will help you to better understand what you need, so you can find who you need. Last but not least, you will learn how to use different tools to resolve your trigger points. Trigger points are a natural occurrence throughout the healing process. They happen because formerly weak and deactivated muscles now are working and getting stronger to support your new movement patterns. At first the muscles will be clumsy and will not coordinate very well, thus creating trigger points. Relieving these trigger points on a day-to-day basis allows for a faster healing process and keeps your muscles happy. Now let's get started on learning how your back works!

LEARNING POINTS FOR CHAPTER 1

1. Back pain is expensive. It has cost the American public an estimated $50 billion. Now that is a lot of money!!!
2. The increases in spinal surgeries and injections to manage chronic back pain have not resulted in an increase in quality of life
3. How you read this book is dependent on your learning style; however, it is recommended after you read a chapter you implement that chapter before going onto the next.
4. If you are impatient (like me), you can read through the entire book once without implementing anything. After you have read the entire book, then take it one chapter at a time. Start with the chapter most interesting to you, and implement each one before going on to the next.

CHAPTER 2

Understanding My Back

The first step to solving back pain is understanding it. Now I am not going to go into a tremendous amount of detail here, not because I cannot or do not want to. I would absolutely love to go into intimate details about the anatomy and paint as clear of a picture for you as possible. However, I do not want your eyes to glaze over, and have you fall out of your chair in absolute boredom. This would likely hurt your back further, which is the complete opposite of my goal for this book. I totally realize, even though anatomy may be absolutely fascinating to me, it is quite likely not for you. So here goes—I am going to keep it simple (promise)...

I want you to put your hands on your hips. Where your hands are located is the wing bones of your pelvis. If you are crazy like me and want the little details – these wing bones are called the ilium – one on the left and one on the right. Your pelvis is made up of three separate bones. Now you know about the first two right? The wing bones—put your hands on your hips again so I know you are following me. Great! Now we are going on to the third bone, which is located directly below your spine. This bone is triangular with a pointy end down. Can you guess what the pointy end is? YES! It is the tailbone. And for you crazies out there who demand the details this bone is called the sacrum.

Now I want you to focus your attention where the triangle bone and the left and right wing bones come together, because it is a very important joint. The reason this joint is important, in my opinion, is because it is the most overlooked and under-treated spot in relation to back pain. I really want you to have a good picture of this joint. If you have to take a break to Google this all-important joint, it is called the sacroiliac joint. I know this is a big word and I do not want to lose you here. So let's try and get a good image in your mind of the sacroiliac joint.

If you Google images of the sacroiliac joint you can see all sorts of good pictures. These will give you a clear picture in your head as we move forward. It is important to have a clear picture in your head because this joint is the foundation of this seven-step system to get rid of your chronic back pain. Again, it is called the sacroiliac joint if you are interested in doing a Google search. However, if a computer is not handy then you can check out what the sacroiliac joint looks like in the picture index at the end of this book.

So why do I consider this sacroiliac joint so important? I know you are wondering this. I equate this joint to the foundation of a house. If the foundation of your house is crooked or uneven, what happens to everything else? You guessed it – doors do not shut right and neither do the windows. In fact, nothing in the house works quite right. The same concept is true with your pelvis. If it is crooked or cattywampus, as I fondly call it, then the spine is stacked on top of it is also not going to work right.

The crooked, or cattywampus positioning of the pelvis causes various painful stress points. Your discs may even end up bulging from the added stress and strain on them. If the discs are stacked up on top of each other the way they are designed to be then they are able to handle stress. However, when they are tilted the strain is too much on them. They can break down and start bulging, causing additional pain for you.

The pelvis is the center balancing point of the body, and there are innumerable muscular attachments to this group of bones. These muscles have difficulty synchronizing themselves when the sacroiliac joint is cattywampus making it hard to support the spine and promote good posture. A large majority of these muscular connections are for the legs and the low back area; however, there is even a connection for a shoulder muscle. For those of you who are curious, it is the latissimus dorsi, which connects at the sacroiliac joint and is a major player in shoulder motion and stabilization. If you do not believe me then go ahead and prove it to yourself. Google "latissimus dorsi." You will see it comes all the way down the back and attaches right on the triangle bone (sacrum) at the sacroiliac joint line. Pretty amazing huh? Puts new meaning to the saying: "The leg bone is attached to the hip bone, the hip bone is connected to the arm bone..." Well you get the point. :-)

You probably are more concerned about the pain going down your legs than your shoulder, right? And rightfully so, because pain radiating down your legs is the pits!!! You may have been told this radiating pain was "sciatica," which is partially true. Sciatica basically means the sciatic nerve is inflamed and irritated. However, this description does not give any indication of why this irritation is happening in the first place. The sciatic nerve does not just start acting up and getting irritated for no reason at all. It is reacting to some sort of pressure somewhere. It is important to understand where this pressure may be coming from that is irritating the sciatic nerve. Okay, I am going to throw another big word at you and I honestly think this is going to be the last one. Here goes—piriformis muscle. Okay, let that word settle in your brain for a second while I help you put the piriformis muscle into this big puzzle called your chronic back pain. In a few moments you will have an understanding of your own personal piriformis muscle.

The pelvis has numerous muscle attachments and the piriformis muscle just happens to be one of them. It is not a big muscle by any means; however, it can be a huge player in back pain. One end actually attaches right at the sacroiliac joint and the other attaches to the hip bone (femur). Of course it makes sense that if the sacroiliac joint is not moving right, this muscle is going to get irritated as well since it attaches right there at the sacroiliac joint.

Unfortunately, when this piriformis muscle gets irritated, it will pinch the sciatic nerve. This pinching occurs because the sciatic nerve goes right through the center of the piriformis muscle before it travels down the leg. Now I am sure you can guess what happens if this piriformis muscle gets unhappy and starts freaking out? You got it—the piriformis muscle squeezes the poor sciatic nerve near to death! This squeezing of the sciatic nerve is why you get all these crazy feelings down the leg—pain, tingling, numbness, feelings of shock. You know exactly what I am talking about. I am sure you have felt all of it before, and quite likely more than once in your life. I know I sure did!

Of course, the poor sciatic nerve will take a further beating after it exits from the piriformis muscle. It is common for the sciatic nerve to get even more irritated at the hamstring muscle, which is located in the back of the thigh or upper leg. The hamstring muscle has two parts, one on the left of the leg and one on the right. The sciatic nerve goes right down the center of them. The hamstring muscle also has tendon attachments at the sacroiliac joint. You know what happens when the sacroiliac joint is not right, don't you? It makes everything else not work right—including the hamstring muscle.

Most of the time the hamstring muscle over-reacts and becomes tight when the sacroiliac joint is off-kilter. As a result, you have this cattywampus sacroiliac joint making the hamstring muscle act erratic and crazy and probably getting tight and miserable. Well, in its misery, the hamstring muscle will yank and pull on the sciatic nerve, thus causing more pain and frustration for you. So here you are with a cattywampus sacroiliac joint, and all these messed up, miserable, and ticked off nerves and muscles. If you at least understood this much, then you are doing very well because this is the basis of what you need to understand. If you are having difficulty getting the details then you are free to read through this last chapter again. It will become more familiar to you as you read it repeatedly. Honestly, all this medical jargon is truly another language so re-reading it will help it settle into your brain a little better.

The main idea you need to take away from this chapter is the sacroiliac joint is the foundation of your body. You want to keep it level and straight so all the other muscles and joints and nerves can do their jobs as they were designed without ticking off each other. I am fully aware medical jargon is not easy to understand. I tried to keep it as simple and lighthearted as possible. I really do not want your eyes glazing over and you falling out of your chair injuring your back even further. That would be bad for all of us. :-)

You may be wondering how exactly I got so involved in understanding this part of the body. I can tell you it definitely was not from school. The approaches taught there for managing sacroiliac joint problems were confusing, so I wanted no part of them. I just happened to go to a 2-for-1 course after I had become a therapist and the "bonus" course was the sacroiliac joint. I volunteered to become a subject on stage so they could correct my problem. I had moderate back pain for years up to that point. To get relief I would have to crack my own lower back and sacroiliac joint. I do not recommend this—it messed me up.

I was completely unprepared for how bad my back really was. Low and behold, they said I was a mess. They did the sacroiliac joint retraining technique and gave me a few exercises to do. I felt an immediate change due to the retraining technique. My whole body felt different. However, I was not prepared for the healing process I would endure to fully resolve the problem.

I had started cracking my back (because it was cool) before my spine had fully matured. Because of this I actually had created a major dysfunction. My body and spine did not know how to stay in the "right" position. My body not knowing the "right" position led to a lot of pain. I had to figure out how to fix it.

I actually had a day where I could not get up off of the floor. It took me about an hour to get up and on numerous days I barely could get out of bed. I have had times where I could not even lift a gallon of milk so I totally get your pain. I know from experience just how terrible and debilitating it can be to have chronic back pain. It seems as though everything in your life revolves around not aggravating the pain.

I honestly never have had a patient with a case as bad as my own. As I learned how to fix my own back problems, I used the tricks and techniques on my patients with fantastic results. Most of the patients who benefit from this approach are women because our hormones make all of our ligaments lax. This allows the pelvis to open up and birth a small bowling ball-sized child. Our hormones also fluctuate through the month, which will affect the flexibility and stability of the ligaments in the spine and pelvis (along with every other ligament and tendon in the body). These changes in ligament flexibility make our bodies more prone to having problems at the sacroiliac joint since there is a tremendous amount of ligamentous support here.

Even though it is most common in women, men are far from immune to the problem. For men, a sacroiliac joint dysfunction usually is preceded by a significant trauma such as a fall, a car accident or impact sports. In some cases a spinal fusion can cause a sacroiliac joint dysfunction since the fusion will force more movement out of the pelvic joints than they were designed to give. (Let's face it, the movement has to occur somewhere).

It honestly did take me years to figure out how to solve this sacroiliac joint problem. I eventually put together an amazing system that really worked using trial and error, with my own pain being a huge motivating factor. All of this experience is put together in a nice little package from which you can benefit.

The first part of the system is getting rid of back spasms. I know you want some sort of relief as quickly as possible, so you will start with some strategies you can use immediately. Then you are going to learn an amazing trick to retrain your back–specifically your pelvis–to move correctly. Next, you need the right muscular support to keep everything moving as it is supposed to move. You will learn just the right exercises to do just that.

The next section deals with the mental-emotional aspect of your back pain. Let's face it, having pain is a very emotional experience. You easily can get stuck there, so you will learn how to free yourself from the mental-emotional experience of pain. Then, you will learn how to relax your muscles with a bodyworker who can help you through the healing process. Last but not least, you will learn how to use tools to manage your own trigger points. I am not going to keep you any longer–I bet you are ready to get to the good stuff and really get rid of your own back pain. So let's keep going!

LEARNING POINTS FOR CHAPTER 2

1. The wing bones of your pelvis are called the ilium. You can find your left and right ilium by placing your hands on your hips.
2. The triangle bone directly below your spine, which also consists of your tailbone, is called the sacrum.
3. The triangle bone and the wing bones create the sacroiliac joint, which is like the foundation of a house. It is important for the sacroiliac joint to be level (not crooked) so the rest of the body can operate properly.
4. The pelvis (including the sacroiliac joint) is the central balancing point of your body.
5. A cattywampus sacroiliac joint can affect your shoulder motion and pain.
6. A cattywampus sacroiliac joint can cause "sciatica," or pain down your leg.
7. The sacroiliac joint is the foundation of your body. You want to keep it level and straight so all the muscles and joints and nerves can do their jobs as they were designed without ticking off each other.
8. Sacroiliac dysfunction is common for women because of our hormones affecting the flexibility and motion at the sacroiliac joint. Men can get sacroiliac joint dysfunction; however, it is usually preceded by a trauma

CHAPTER 3

Eliminate Back Spasms!

You have back pain, and maybe it is even chronic back pain, so I am quite certain you are miserable. It may feel like a screwdriver is being driven into your back. It makes everything "lock up." You cannot move out of a certain position until it releases. Back spasms are no joke–they are downright debilitating. They make sleeping and even moving difficult. These painful spasms can stop you in your tracks no matter what you are doing. Luckily, I have a few strategies you can use to help alleviate your back spasms, and maybe even prevent them in the first place.

The first strategy I will give you is magnesium. Yes it is that simple–just magnesium. It is not some outrageously expensive item you have to sell your left arm to get. It is estimated more than fifty percent of the U.S. population does not get their recommended daily intake for magnesium and that is on the conservative side. It is likely eighty percent of the U.S. population is deficient. There are several good reasons for this deficiency and I will address a few with you right now.

First and foremost, magnesium comes from leafy green veggies, which presents an issue for individuals who do not like to eat their veggies. Magnesium also comes from the husk of the wheat germ, which is processed out while making white bread and other common foods.

Magnesium deficiency is further compounded when magnesium is not in the soil to begin with. When the mineral is not in the soil then it can't be taken up by the plant growing in that soil. Then, obviously it is not in your food.

I want you to be aware that even though I am focusing on magnesium, I am not saying all the other vitamins are not important. Your body is only as healthy as what you put in it and if your body is unhealthy then it is going to hurt. Good nutrition is important and the whole conversation about nutrition is much too large to cover in this book.

The basic rule I incorporate with nutrition is: If it came from the earth, then your body knows what to do with it. If the food was processed by machines, then your body is unable to readily recognize the nutrition in the food, and cannot utilize it properly. So the closer your food is to the natural form from the earth, then the higher nutritional value it will have for your body.

Coming back from the tangent, let's get back to magnesium. Magnesium has numerous important benefits to your body; however, I am only going to focus on one with you today. Magnesium is a natural muscle relaxer. It also helps relax the nervous system. This is important because it will help relax your muscles and your body while at rest and during sleep.

To give you a deeper understanding of how magnesium works on the body, four minerals present in your muscle cells are responsible for properly contracting your muscles. These four minerals are magnesium, calcium, potassium and sodium. Without going into the boring details, magnesium is responsible for getting the muscle cells to chill out and relax.

It is interesting to note calcium does just the opposite. It excites the muscle cells, thus causing the muscles to tighten and contract. There is a big effort to increase awareness of calcium deficiency, which can cause weak bones. So more people such as yourself are taking more calcium supplements. Taking more calcium for strong bones is a great idea. However, if the body has too much calcium present relative to the magnesium that will make your muscles chronically tight, which leads to soreness, spasms and pain. Nobody needs or wants that; especially you when you are trying to manage your back pain already.

Magnesium can be used on a daily basis just to keep your muscles calmed down, which will then will keep your pain down as well. The extra relaxation in your muscles will allow you to chill out and relax better and also give you a better night's sleep. Another great way to utilize magnesium is taking an additional dose if you do something to pull or strain your back. That will prevent strong muscle spasms that will debilitate you for the remainder of the day.

A great example of taking magnesium as a preventative measure is the day I was mowing the grass and stepped in a hole. I felt the pull in my back. Although it did not hurt right away, I knew it was likely it would hurt later since I could feel the pull right at my lower back.

I decided to shut off the mower, go inside, and take a large dose of magnesium to prevent any spasms from stopping me later in the day. It worked. I felt some mild stiffness at the end of the day and a little the next morning but no spasms and no unrelenting pain preventing me from doing what I wanted with my day. I successfully prevented my body from going into a spasm pain cycle.

You even can put magnesium oil on your skin that will absorb into the body and affect that specific area. For example, you can put the oil on your back and calm down that specific area. It is great to use if you really want to target a certain area of your body such as your lower back and hip areas.

Another way to get magnesium into your system is through an age-old remedy–the Epsom salts bath. Epsom salts are really just magnesium sulfate. When you place the salts into a hot bath and soak in the mixture, your skin's pores open up from the heat and the magnesium sulfate will absorb into your body and relax your muscles. There is no better way to comfort and nurture yourself than with an Epsom salts bath–and it is healthy for you and your muscles.

As a bonus, if you take an Epsom salts bath at the end of the day, right before going to sleep, falling asleep will be easier for two reasons. One is the magnesium will help your muscles relax since it is a muscle relaxer. The second is as your body cools down, it naturally gets sleepy, which is the perfect time to get some good, quality sleep.

Maybe the easiest way to get additional magnesium into your body is through supplements. A lot of supplements available on the market. You need to be aware not all of them are created equal. Originally, magnesium is present as a rock in the ground and, last time I checked, your body could not digest "rocks". Therefore, be aware of what you are purchasing, because some of the cheapest forms may not be digestible.

A company called Cardiovascular Research Ltd. has the best magnesium I have found so far. Please note, I have not tried all the products out there. I actually have not tried too many since once I find something that works for me I do not keep trying other kinds. I have tried a handful of others and found they did not compare. I ended up going back to using the Cardiovascular Research Ltd. and have not tried anything afterward.

In your experience, some other highly effective and wonderful brands may be super effective for your body and that is great. I just happened to have settled with Cardiovascular Research Ltd. because it works for me and many others to whom I have recommended it. I have found Cardiovascular Research Ltd.'s supplements to be easily absorbable and cost effective as well.

In general, when purchasing magnesium, the liquid forms tend to be faster acting than the capsules. So be aware of that if you want a faster acting form of magnesium. Occasionally, magnesium can have a negative effect on your intestines (it can loosen those muscles, too). In those instances, I have found taking additional vitamin C helps alleviate that.

The next strategy used to decrease muscle spasms is completely free. Yes, you got it—free. It will not cost you a dime or a penny or even a nickel. Even better than that, you can use this strategy anywhere—in the bathroom, on a plane, in the car—you just name it. This strategy is breathing—yes *breathing*. Indeed, breathing is a simple concept; however, effective breathing is worth its weight in gold. Let me explain my rationale on this, so we are both on the same page.

When you are in pain, it is likely you take short, shallow breaths. This tends to be a very common pain reaction, but unfortunately, when you take those shallow breaths it also excites the part of your nervous system responsible for your fight-or-flight reaction. So what happens when your muscles are preparing to fight something or run away from danger? You are right—they tighten up. If your muscles tighten up then that will increase your pain byincreasing your muscle spasms.

So, it is as simple as that—shallow breathing increases the fight-or-flight response and your cortisol levels. That makes your muscles tight and increases your spasms, which is something you definitely do not want. Incorporating some good breathing techniques is going to help you relax and rest when it is time to rest, get rid of muscle spasms and decrease your pain. So let's learn how to incorporate some good breathing techniques to alleviate this fight-or-flight pain spasm cycle.

First of all, you need to just get used to taking as much air as possible into your lungs. You should feel your lungs fill up as full as possible, and allow your ribs to expand as far as they will go. You may even feel stretching in the muscles attached to your ribcage.

If your body is not used to getting so much oxygen, you may notice you get lightheaded after a few breaths. That is okay, and totally normal. It is nothing to worry about; however, if it bothers you stop until the lightheaded feeling goes away then try again. Eventually, when you do the deep breathing you no longer will notice the lightheadedness because your body will be used to getting all that oxygen again.

Now I want you to take the deep breathing one step further. You know how when you finish with a long day at work or finish a stressful project you sit down and breathe a sigh of relief? Remember how good it feels to the body as you breathe that sigh of relief because it drains the stress right out of your muscles? Basically, when you break down the mechanics, a sigh is just an exhale that is a bit longer than the inhale.

It is easy to incorporate a "sigh-like" breathing pattern to help alleviate stress, decrease muscle tightness and turn off "fight or flight" reaction. The way to incorporate a "sigh like" breathing pattern is taking the time to inhale for three full seconds and then exhaling for a full four seconds.

If you have big lungs shoot for a five second inhale and a seven second exhale. You should notice immediately how it allows your muscles to relax and your body to calm down overall. This will make it easier for you to rest and sleep. It is likely you will notice your pain level drop a notch or two from maybe a seven out of ten to maybe a five or six out of ten. This is pretty impressive since it is free, simple and even portable—you can do it anywhere!

The next strategy requires something you likely already have in your cupboard: ibuprofen, which is generic for Advil and naproxen, which is generic for Aleve. Both of these are NSAIDS (non-steroidal anti-inflammatory drugs), which are great for targeting your body's muscular system a bit better than Tylenol or aspirin. Both ibuprofen and naproxen will help get rid of pain, especially if it is related to inflammation. They are specifically used to alleviate inflammation.

If you are interested in finding more natural anti-inflammatory solutions then you have several choices. Bromelain comes from the pineapple and in concentrated capsule form is a natural anti-inflammatory. It is relatively inexpensive but may be difficult to find in some health food stores. However, I have found it is easy to find online with a good Google search or on Amazon.

It can be nice to get a blend of different ingredients to get a more effective natural anti-inflammatory. Two products I am aware of on the market use a blend of ingredients. One is called Zyflamend and the other is Wobenzym. Both are great products; however, they can be a bit on the expensive side.

The benefit to taking these supplements is they are not hard on the liver, kidneys or stomach like such ibuprofen and naproxen. This means you do not have to worry about taking them in higher dosages. You may even combine the NSAIDS with the natural anti-inflammatories for an added punch when you need it without worrying about damaging your body's organs.

Now that we are on the topic of anti-inflammatories I am going to take you into the realm of what you can use on your skin that will be absorbed and affect the muscles beneath them. You already learned about magnesium oil, which can be placed on the skin as a natural muscle relaxer; however, it is great to have a product with anti-inflammatory, pain relief and muscle relaxant properties. This differs from the icy hot products you see in the stores because their purpose is to distract the nerves of the body from the pain. The Icy Hot pain relief products usually do little for the actual muscle spasm or inflammation.

One company I have found with products addressing inflammation, pain and tight muscles is called Peaceful Mountain, Inc. I have used and recommended most of their products consistently without disappointment. My favorite products tend to be Joint Rescue, Back and Neck Rescue and Muscle Rescue.

Joint Rescue is my primary go-to product because it is a strong anti-inflammatory that includes the herb devil's claw. Joint Rescue also helps address pain relief with white willow and arnica. Back and Neck Rescue is a great product because it helps calm down nerve pain and inflammation with the herb St. John's wort. Back and Neck Rescue also addresses pain relief with arnica and white willow while decreasing spasms with lavender.

Muscle Rescue is another great product and it is based upon homeopathy. I also have found this homeopathic remedy to be great for getting soreness out of muscles. Any of these products would be great to help you decrease your back pain. If you want to see a full line of Peaceful Mountain Inc.'s products you can go to their website www.peacefulmountain.com and see what they have to offer.

LEARNING POINTS FOR CHAPTER 3
1. It is likely eighty percent of the U.S. population is deficient in magnesium.
2. Magnesium is a natural muscle relaxer.
3. Magnesium oil placed on your skin will help with relaxing the muscles in the area.
4. Epsom salts (which are magnesium sulfate) can be used in a bath to relax your muscles.
5. Magnesium is a very cost effective supplement, and the liquid form may absorb more quickly into your body than the capsules
6. Shallow breathing increases your "fight or flight" reaction and your cortisol levels.
7. Incorporating a sigh-like breathing pattern will help reverse your "fight or flight" reaction.
8. Natural anti-inflammatories are a great way to get rid of inflammation without damaging other organs of your body and can complement traditional NSAIDS nicely.
9. Peaceful Mountain Inc. makes some great all natural gels you can place on your skin to address inflammation, muscle spasms and pain.

CHAPTER 4

Retrain Your Back to Move Right

Now that you can decrease your back spasms using several strategies I want to address the reason why the spasms are there in the first place. If your sacroiliac joint is not working properly, then it can be an underlying cause of back spasms and, of course, pain.

If you remember back to the beginning of the book, you will recall the anatomy lesson. While learning about your back's anatomy you learned all about the sacroiliac joint. You learned about some of the different muscles attaching there such as the latissimus dorsi, the piriformis and the hamstring–which, of course, are only a small portion of the muscles that attach there; however, they are some of the major players in your back pain.

I do not want to go into great detail on all the muscles attaching to the pelvis and lower back region. I am making a conscious effort to keep this as simple as possible for you. If you do not remember the sacroiliac joint then I would recommend you scan back through that section before going any further in this section. You also can find a few pictures of the sacroiliac joint in the Picture Index at the end of the book.

It is quite important you have a basic understanding of anatomy here. Now you are going to learn how to re-educate your sacroiliac joint so it will move properly for you and keep the muscles supported by your pelvis happy. You may even want to have a picture of the sacroiliac joint as a reference as you learn about the next steps in re-educating your sacroiliac joint.

A subtle movement occurs at the sacroiliac joint during both back and hip motions. This motion occurs when you flex your spine forward and extend it backward. Even while the hip flexes up toward your chest and extends behind you, you have movement at your sacroiliac joint. The triangle bone in the center (sacrum) moves up and slightly forward during all of these movements. Now, what I have discovered is many times this triangle bone is going the opposite direction or it is not moving at all. So it needs a gentle "nudge" to re-educate or re-train it and get it moving in the right direction again.

You are going to learn how to do this simple technique in easy-to-follow steps. The only problem you may have is finding a partner to help with this re-training technique. Your partner is going to push and give your bones a gentle "nudge" while you move your body in specificpositions to retrain the joint.

You are going to stand up with your feet about hip width apart, with your weight spread as evenly as you can between the two feet. If you need support, then have a chair back or table in front of you to lean on. Your partner is going to be sitting directly next to you. He or she will place one palm on the front of your wing bone (the ilium) and the other hand will be placed on the triangle bone (sacrum).

If you are uncertain of the placement of the hands then you can refer to the pictures located one paragraph down. The hand on the wing bone is going to be pushing backward and the hand on the triangle bone is going to be pushing forward. Basically, your partner is going to be encouraging proper joint movement and retraining the sacroiliac joint to move as it is supposed to move.

Remember there are two sacroiliac joints, one on the left and one on the right. Therefore, they have to push on the wing bone on the left and the wing bone on the right for each of the movements. The palm of the back hand will be placed on the triangle bone keeping it slightly shifted to the side you are working on without having your palm on the sacroiliac joint itself. If you are uncertain, just keep the palm in the center. Your partner only has to push with fifteen to twenty pounds of pressure between both hands to effectively retrain your sacroiliac joint.

The first retraining movement is the forward bending position. To do this you are going to bend forward while your partner is holding fifteen to twenty pounds of pressure between both hands. You bend as far forward as you can and then come back up to a straight position. Refer to the pictures below for proper hand placement. As soon as you stand back up to a straight position, then your partner can release their fifteen to twenty pounds of pressure and both of you can relax. You are going to repeat this three times on each side before you go onto the next retraining movement.

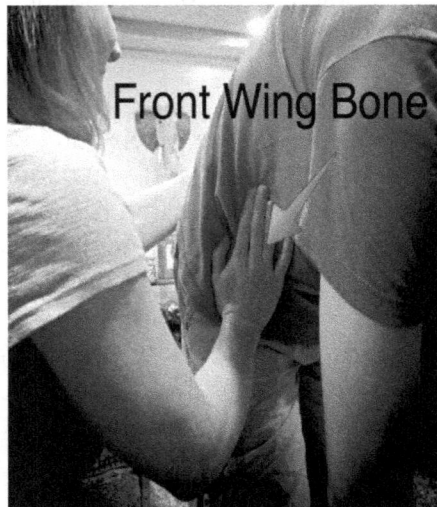

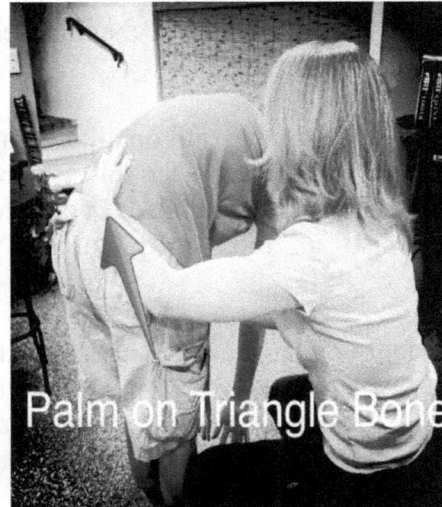

The second retraining movement backward bending. For this movement it is going to be similar to the first except instead of bending forward, you are going to be leaning backward with your back. So again, make sure your feet are about shoulder width apart with your weight evenly distributed.

Your partner is going to push with about fifteen to twenty pounds of pressure with one hand on the wing bone and the other on the triangle bone. Refer to the pictures below if you are uncertain of the hand placements. While your partner is exerting the fifteen to twenty pounds of pressure, you are going to lean back as far as you can while holding onto something (if needed for support and balance).

After you go back as far as you possibly can without falling backward, then come back up to a straightened position. Once you get to a straightened position your partner can release their fifteen to twenty pounds of pressure on the triangle and wing bones.

Repeat this movement three times with the pressure on each side of the sacroiliac joint. Remember, your partner is going to be pushing on the right wing bone three times and then the left wing bone three times. The back hand is always placed on the triangle bone in the center, keeping a slight shift to the side of the sacroiliac joint you are working.

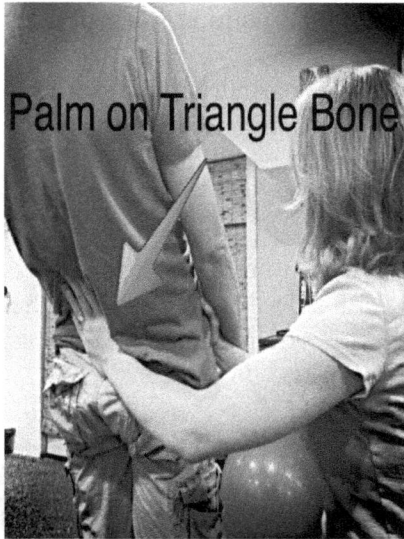
Palm on Triangle Bone

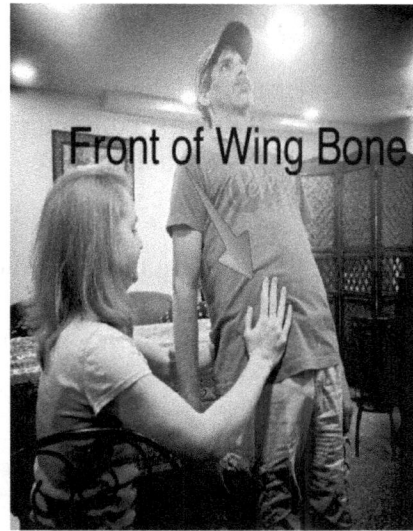
Front of Wing Bone

The third retraining movement is flexing your hip up to your stomach, also considered bringing your knee to your chest. During this movement you definitely will need something to hold onto since you are going to be standing on one leg and it can be easy to lose your balance.

Start with shifting your weight off to the opposite side before your partner starts pushing on your pelvis. Once you feel you have your balance, your partner can start pushing fifteen to twenty pounds of pressure on the triangle bone and the wing bone. Meanwhile you lift your knee up to your chest as far as you can and then bring it back down to the floor. Once your foot is securely placed on the floor then your partner can release the pressure on your pelvis.

This is repeated three times on each side. Whatever side you are pushing on is the side you are lifting your knee up for. For example, say your partner is pushing on your right wing bone in the front so you are going to lift your right knee up to your chest.

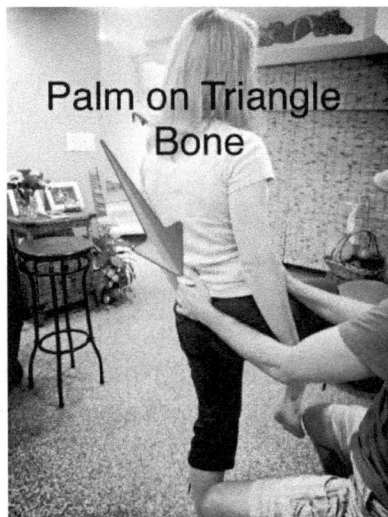
Palm on Triangle Bone

The fourth and final retraining movement is the hip extension or back-kick of the leg. Once again you are going to be standing on one leg, so it is advised to hold onto something for support of your balance.

Start by shifting your weight off to the opposite side before your partner starts pushing on your pelvis. Once you have your balance established, your partner can start pushing fifteen to twenty pounds of pressure on your pelvis while you kick your leg back as far as you can then bring it back down to the floor.

Once your foot is securely placed on the floor then your partner can release the pressure on your pelvis and both of you can relax. This is repeated three times on each side just as it was for the knee to chest movement. Whatever side your partner is pushing on is the side you are back kicking with your leg.

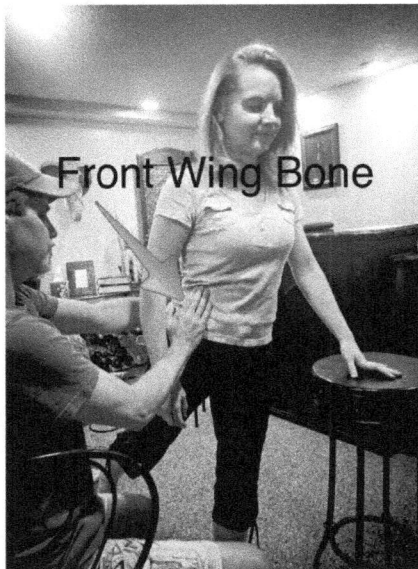

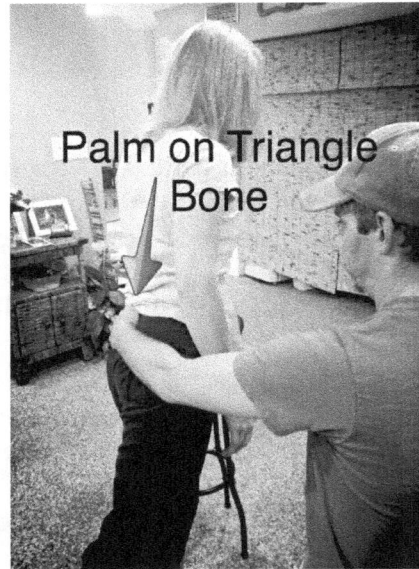

Most certainly you want to do this whole routine on both sides. To make it easier for you to reference the steps are given in an easy-to-follow format below:

Forward Bending
Keep feet shoulder width apart
Keep weight evenly distributed between both feet
Partner sits at one side
Partner places one palm on triangle bone and the other palm on front wing bone
Partner pushes with fifteen to twenty pounds of pressure and holds this pressure through your movement
Hold on to a chair or table for safety if necessary
Bend forward as far as you can and then come back up straight
Once you are completely straight up then your partner releases the pressure
Repeat three times on each side

Backward Bending
Keep feet shoulder width apart
Keep weight evenly distributed between both feet
Partner sits at one side
Partner places one palm on the triangle bone and the other palm on front wing bone
Partner pushes with fifteen to twenty pounds pressure and holds this pressure through your movement
Hold on to a chair or table for safety if necessary
Bend forward as far as you can and then come back up straight
Once you are completely straight up then your partner releases the pressure
Repeat three times on each side

Knee to Chest
Partner sits at one side
Partner places one palm on the triangle bone and the other palm on the wing bone
Shift your weight to the opposite side
Partner starts pushing with fifteen to twenty pounds of pressure and holds this pressure through your movement
Hold onto a chair or table for safety
Bring your hip up with your knee towards your chest as far as you can
Place your foot securely back on the ground and then your partner can release their pressure
Repeat this three times on each side

Hip Extension or Back Kick
Partner sits at one side
Partner places one palm on the triangle bone and the other palm on the wing bone
Shift your weight to the opposite side
Partner starts pushing with fifteen to twenty pounds of pressure and holds this pressure through your movement
Hold onto a chair or table for safety
Kick your leg back as far as you can
Place your foot securely back on the ground and then your partner can release their pressure
Repeat this three times on each side

After this is done you will notice an immediate change in your back, with increased range of motion and a decreased tenseness or pressure in your back and, hopefully, decreased pain as well. If you are lucky, it only will take one time doing this to get the joint and muscles trained to move properly. However, if you are like most individuals (me included), you may need it done a few times a week to keep everything lined up.

Once the joints, ligaments and soft tissues get used to the new positioning, they will hold on their own;

however, it can take weeks or months for this to happen. In my experience the length of time you had a back dysfunction (in years) determines the amount of months it will take to heal. Therefore if you had a back issue for ten years it will take ten months to sort it out and get the joints, ligaments, tendons and soft tissues used to the new placement. I urge you to be patient with this process and trust that it will heal. Again, I know how frustrating this process is first-hand because I also wanted results yesterday. Getting frustrated will not help your healing process. So take some deep breaths and just allow the process to happen and trust in your body's ability to heal itself.

I also recommend using a sacroiliac support belt to facilitate this process after the retraining procedure is completed. This belt is an everyday use support belt that will keep the sacroiliac joint lined up properly. It may take several months for the healing process to complete, and using the sacroiliac belt will help speed up this process and make it more comfortable.

If you have a sacroiliac belt then go ahead and use what you have. If you do not have one already then I would recommend getting one from Serola. I have personally used this belt and find it to be comfortable and easy to wear under clothing. It is unobtrusive and most importantly IT WORKS! It does exactly what it is supposed to in keeping the joint lined up properly to further facilitate retraining and support of the joint and surrounding muscles.

It is important to keep the sacroiliac joint lined up properly because the more the joints, ligaments, tendons, muscles and soft tissue are placed in the new proper position, the more quickly they will accept their new place. To get a Serola sacroiliac belt go to the website www.serola.net. You will find instructions on the site so you can order the correct size for your body.

LEARNING POINTS FOR CHAPTER 4

1. A subtle movement occurs at your sacroiliac joint with all hip motion and front and back bending of the spine.
2. Using a partner you are going to give the sacroiliac joint a gentle "nudge" to move it the way it is supposed to move.
3. Your partner is going to place one hand on the triangle bone and the other on the front of the wing bone. Then he or she will push the palms toward each other for each of the movements to retrain the sacroiliac joint.
4. Use of a sacroiliac belt after the retraining movements may help with your healing process and make it more comfortable.
5. It may take months for the healing process to complete. As a rule of thumb the amount of years the problem has been there is how many months it will take to heal (for example five years = five months)

CHAPTER 5

Muscular Support

At this point you need to know what to do to develop the right muscles for supporting the area of the spine and the pelvis. This is where the work really begins for you. The muscles supporting the spine and pelvis are all part of the "core" of your body. These muscles lend support and strength to everything you do. The crazy thing is I historically have found the core muscles are the weakest muscles for the majority of my clients and patients who are suffering from back pain.

When the sacroiliac joint is not moving correctly, many of the muscles responsible for your core strength are shut down or deactivated so they cannot contract fully. They may only be able to operate at partial capacity. Now that you have done the retraining exercise and you are wearing the sacroiliac belt from Serola, you are ready to wake up these core muscles. Then they can support your back and pelvis the way they were designed to do.

Before you learn the nitty gritty of the specific exercises you need to support and heal from your chronic back pain, you first need to become familiar with one of your major core muscles in the front of your belly. It is called the transverse abdominus muscle (sorry, another big word), which functions like a corset or a back brace keeping the abdominal area rigid and strong.

You are invited to Google the transverse abdominus muscle so you can get an adequate picture in your mind. It is totally okay to stop for a minute or two and look up this muscle. As you can see, this muscle attaches from one wing bone (ilium) to the other wing bone (ilium) and spans the space between the pelvis and the ribcage. The fibers of this muscle go horizontally, which means when it contracts it pulls all of your abdominal contents inward.

A beautiful bonus with exercising this muscle is when it is tone and fit, it can help reduce your waist by inches. Truly, I have had numerous patients and clients tell me they had not lost weight from the exercises; however, they lost inches on their waist and were able to wear a smaller size pant. If you happen to be vain as I am then you will really appreciate this bonus :-)

It is time for you to find this muscle on your own body. I want you to put your hands on your hips with your fingers resting in front. Your fingers should be resting right on the front of your wing bones (ilium). Bring your fingers toward the center just slightly, maybe only an inch or so, until they sink into the soft belly area. This is where it is easiest to feel the contraction of that corset muscle (transverse abdominus).

The corset muscle (transverse abdominus) automatically contracts when you either cough or sneeze. Since you cannot consciously sneeze then let's take the route of doing a fake cough. With your fingers placed right on soft spot just to the inside of the wing bones I want you to fake a good hearty cough. You will feel the soft spot harden a little and maybe even pull inward toward your spine.

You likely have been completely unaware of this muscle being there unless you got a bad cold and were coughing all the time. You got sore in your belly and that was the corset muscle (transverse abdominus). Up until now this muscle has been contracting and doing its job unconsciously. It is kind of like a wild horse–it does what it wants when it wants. Now it is time for you to take the reins and tell the horse what to do.

Consciously pull your belly in and try to feel for the same contraction you had when you faked a cough. Please be patient with yourself! This wild horse may not be easily tamed so just keep working at it. You can keep doing a fake cough until you can consciously figure out how to get the corset muscle (transverse abdominus) to activate. This may take a few minutes or a few days, so no worries and take your time. This concept is a foundation for all ten exercises you are going to learn shortly. Once you gain conscious control of this muscle then you can work on contracting this muscle at any time such as when you are sitting in your car, or standing in one place while making dinner.

I need to cover one more thing before you learn the different exercises. I want to cover the concept of what these exercises may feel like. These exercises may be a bit uncomfortable to do initially. There may be sensations of pulling in different muscles and areas and that is completely acceptable and even desirable. There may be even some increase in pain with some of the exercises.

A mild to moderate pain increase is acceptable, and for the majority of people, as more repetitions are done the discomfort tends to decrease. However, if the discomfort is sharp or pain increase is severe then hold off on that specific exercise for maybe a week. Then try it again and see if it feels better. Your body may not be strong enough or prepared to do exercises yet and that is okay. Please honor what your body is telling you. Now let's get started with the exercises:

Pelvic Tilt or simply called the Tummy Tuck

Lie on your back on the bed or floor
Bend your knees up and keep your feet flat on the bed or floor
Activate and tighten your corset (transverse abdominus) muscle
Pull your belly in toward your spine and flatten your back into the bed or floor
Hold for one to three seconds then relax
Repeat ten to thirty repetitions depending on fatigue

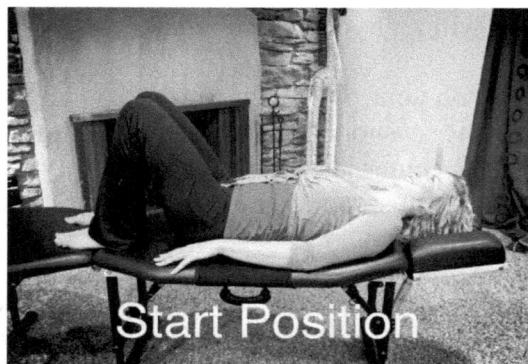
Start Position

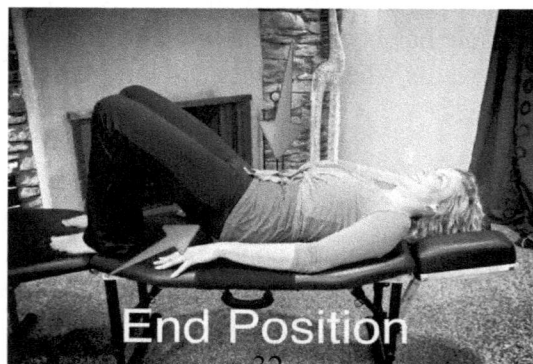
End Position

Bridging

Lie on your back on the bed or floor
Bend your knees up and keep your feet flat on the bed or floor
Place a pillow (folded to make it a bit thicker) or a six to ten inch ball between your knees
Hold the pillow or ball in place with mild to moderate pressure
Activate and tighten your corset (transverse abdominus) muscle
Push through your heels and lift your buttocks off of the bed or floor as high as you can comfortably
Hold lifted position for two to three seconds then slowly lower back down and relax for one second
Repeat ten to thirty repetitions depending on fatigue

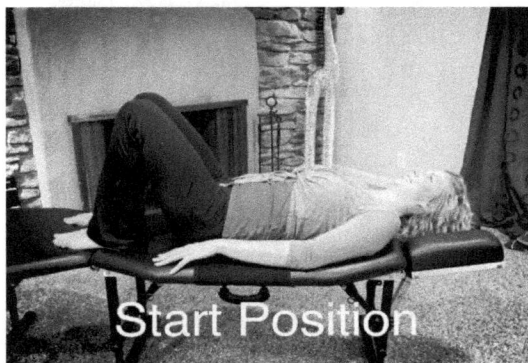
Start Position

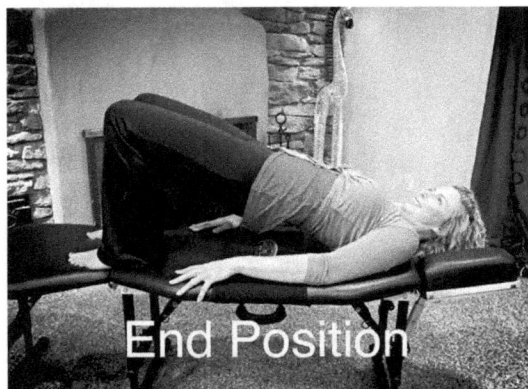
End Position

<u>Press Up on Belly</u>

Lie flat on your stomach
Come up to your elbows
Inhale as deeply as you can
As you completely exhale then activate and tighten your corset (transverse abdominus) muscle
You will feel with the exhale the spine relaxing down into the position
Lower yourself back down flat to the bed or the floor
Repeat ten to thirty repetitions depending on fatigue

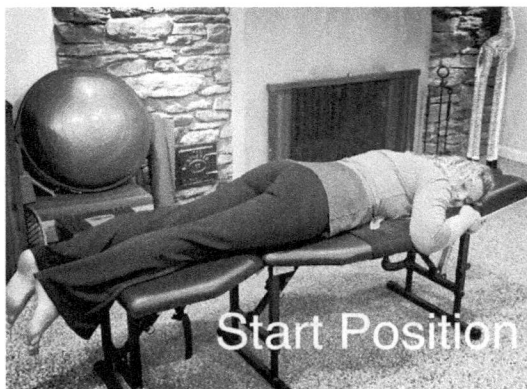

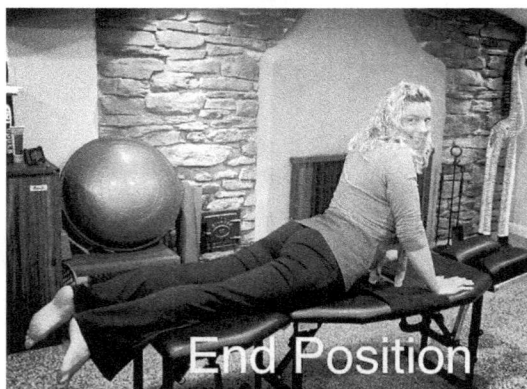

Back Kick on Belly

Lie flat on your stomach
Rest your arms under your chin to support your neck and head or place under your forehead
Activate and tighten your corset (transverse abdominus) muscle
Keep your knee locked straight
Lift your heel up toward the ceiling as far as is comfortable for you
Hold for one to three seconds then slowly lower back down and relax
Repeat ten to thirty repetitions depending on fatigue

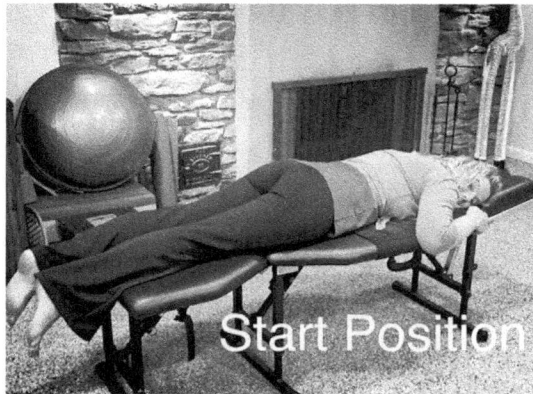

Start Position

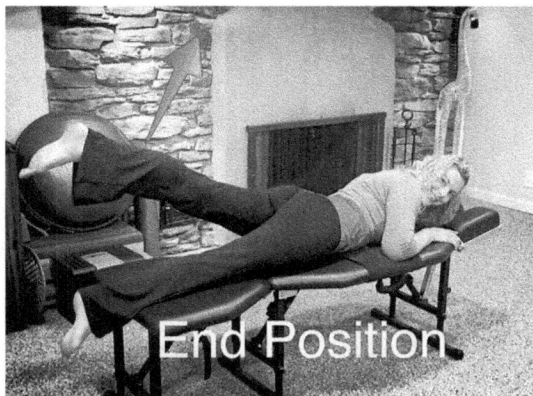

End Position

Scissor kick

Lie on your side
Keep your hips stacked on top of one another
Avoid rolling forward or backward with the top hip
Support your head and neck with the bottom arm or shoulder
Activate and tighten your corset (transverse abdominus) muscle
Lift your leg straight in the air as high as is comfortable
Keep the knee and toes pointed forward, bringing the outer ankle toward the ceiling
Hold for one to two seconds then slowly lower back down and relax
Repeat ten to thirty repetitions depending on fatigue

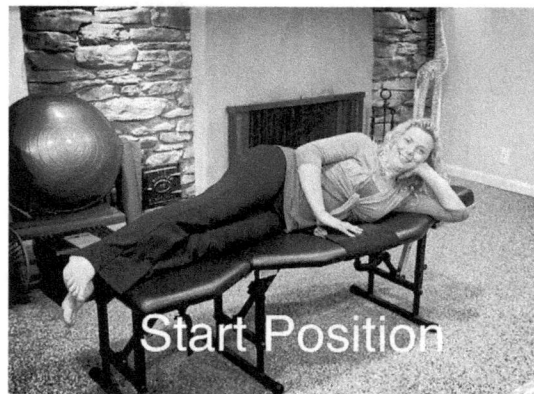

Start Position

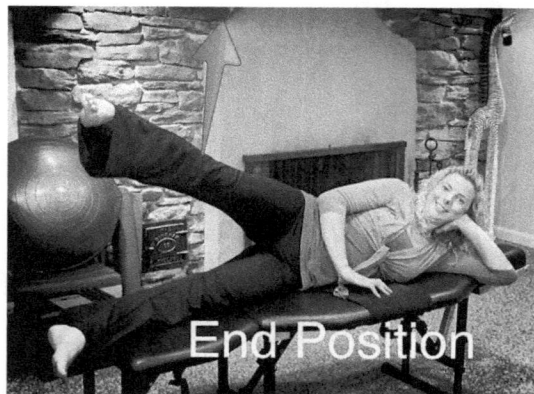

End Position

Pigeon Toe Exercise

Lie flat on your back OR long-sit on the bed or floor with your legs in front, knees straight
Keep your feet about shoulder-width apart
Activate and tighten your corset (transverse abdominus) muscle
Roll your legs inward so your big toes are trying to touch
Basically you are putting yourself into a pigeon toe position
Hold the pigeon toe position for one to three seconds and slowly release and relax
Repeat ten to thirty repetitions depending on fatigue

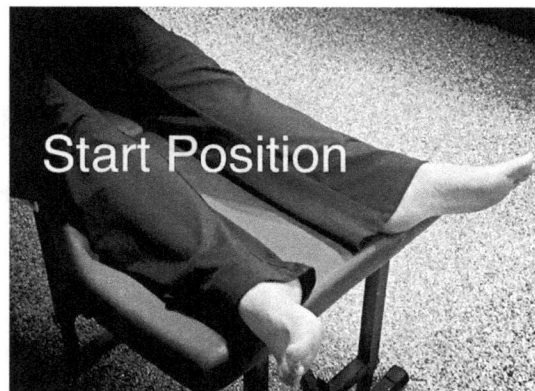

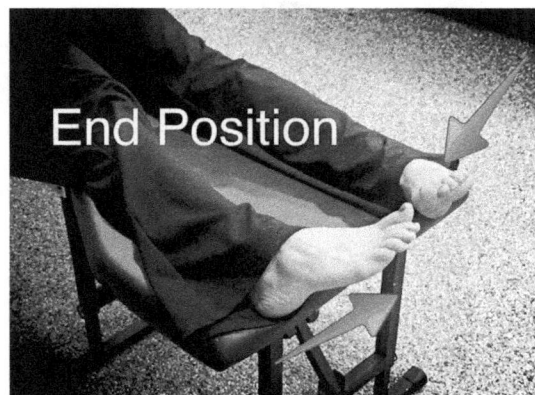

Knee Bend Hip Drop

Stand straight with feet about shoulder-width apart
Activate and tighten your corset (transverse abdominus) muscle
Lock one knee straight and bend the other knee
Keep both heels on the floor
The knee is bending, the hip will drop slightly
You will feel movement occurring in your back right at the sacroiliac joint
Straighten and lock the bent knee
Bend the opposite knee and allow the hip to drop slightly
Alternate sides, creating reciprocal movement at the sacroiliac joint
Repeat ten to thirty repetitions depending on fatigue

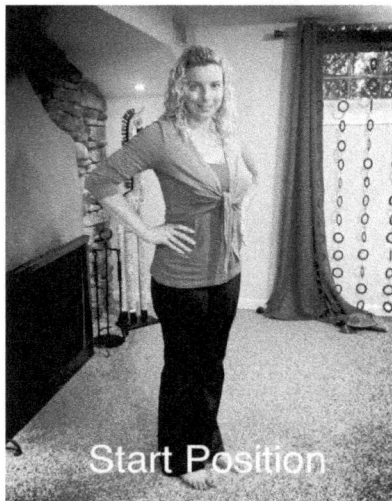

Start Position

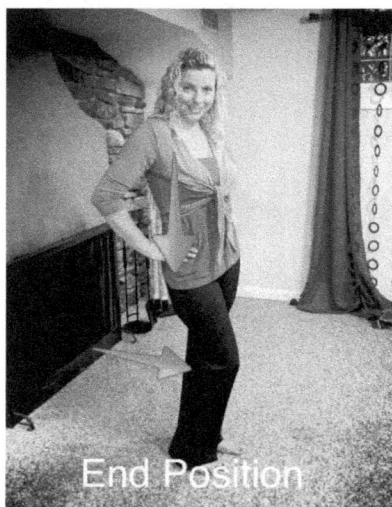

End Position

Isometric Hip Exercise

Stand with your feet about hip-width apart
Keep your feet in this position
Tighten your muscles as though you are pulling your feet in toward one another
Tighten and hold this pulling for three to five seconds then relax
Rest for one to two seconds
Tighten your muscles as though you are pushing your feet apart
Tighten and hold this pushing for three to five seconds then relax
Rest for one to two seconds
Cycle between pulling in and pushing out
Repeat ten to thirty repetitions depending on fatigue

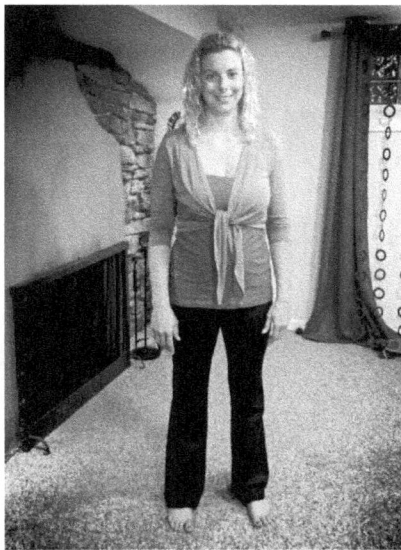

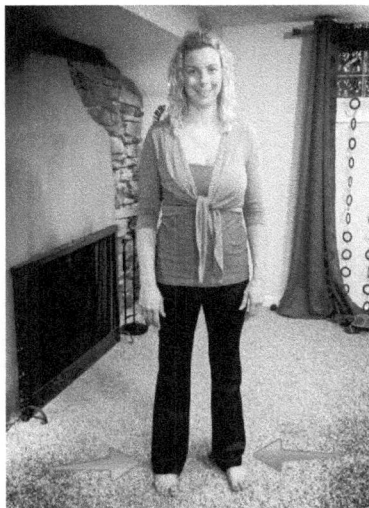
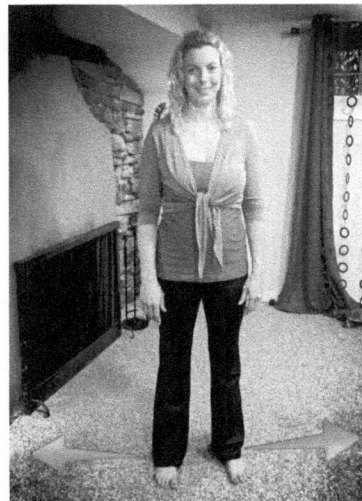

Seated Sidebend

Sit comfortably on the edge of your bed or couch
Keep your hips and knees at approximately a ninety-degree angle
Activate and tighten your corset (transverse abdominus) muscle
Bend your elbows so your hand is near shoulder level
Lean over to the side bringing your elbow down next to your hip
Keep both of your butt bones touching the bed or couch
Hold for one to two seconds and then slowly come back up to a straightened position
Lean over to the opposite side bringing your elbow down next to your hip
Keep both of your butt bones touching the bed or couch
Hold for one to two seconds then slowly come back up to a straightened position
Alternate sides
Repeat ten to thirty repetitions to each side depending on fatigue

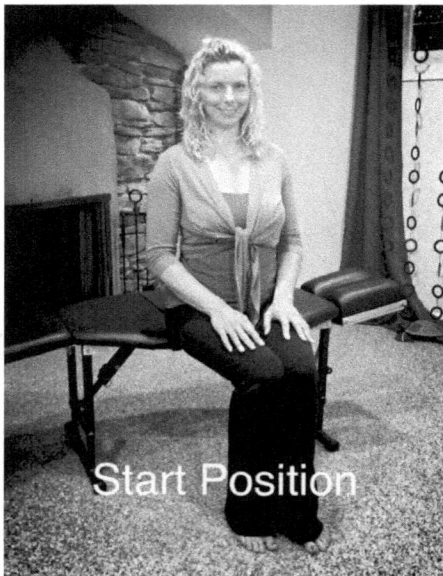

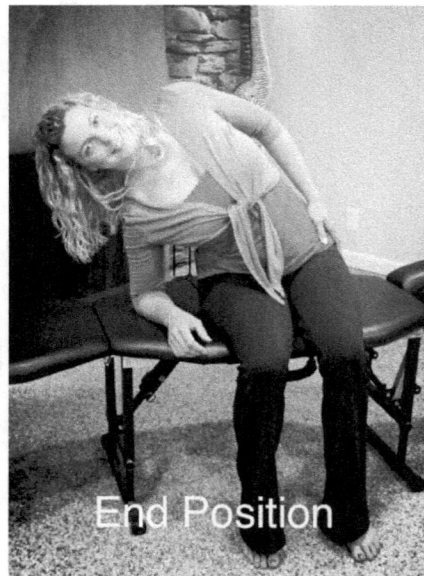

Start Position

End Position

Hamstring Stretch

Sit on the edge of a chair, couch or bed
Make certain your butt bones are right on the edge of the seat
Straighten out one leg with the knee fully locked out
Keep the heel of the fully straightened knee on the floor
Keep the whole foot of the bent and supporting leg flat on the floor
Activate and tighten your corset (transverse abdominus) muscle
Lean forward leading with the chest and not the shoulders
Lean forward until the point where you feel a stretch in the straightened leg
Stretch should be felt in the backside of the straightened leg
Hold this stretch position for thirty seconds then bend the knee back and place the foot flat

Repeat on the other side

Straighten out one leg with the knee fully locked out
Keep the heel of the fully straightened knee on the floor
Keep the whole foot of the bent and supporting leg flat on the floor
Activate and tighten your corset (transverse abdominus) muscle
Lean forward leading with the chest and not the shoulders
Lean forward until the point where you feel a stretch in the straightened leg
Hold this position for thirty seconds then bend the knee back and place the foot flat
Repeat three on each side

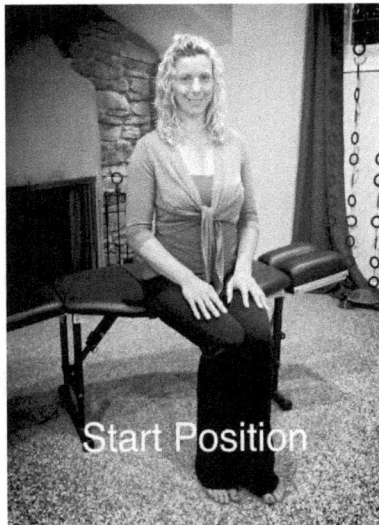

Start Position

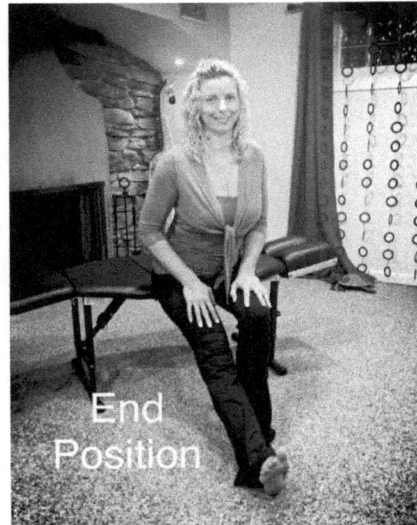

End Position

All of the above exercises play an important role in supporting the pelvis and the spine. You may not be able to do all of them initially. Work your way into being able to do each of the exercises fully. Listen to your body and hear what it is saying to you.

There may be exercises that feel better than others and you may notice more benefit from those as well. Put those particular exercises on the top of the priority list and make certain you do not miss them. You may even want to do those particular exercises multiple times a day. All of the exercises should be done daily. If you are wanting to do only ten repetitions at a time, you can do the exercises two times a day to get more benefit.

LEARNING POINTS FOR CHAPTER 5

1. The muscles supporting the spine and pelvis are all part of the "core" of your body.
2. The core muscles are the weakest muscles for the majority of individuals who are suffering from back pain.
3. The retraining exercise in Chapter 4 and use of the sacroiliac belt helps to "wake up" your core muscles.
4. The corset muscle (transverse abdominus) is the foundation of your core muscles.
5. When you fake a cough you will feel your abdomen tighten and pull in–this is the corset muscle.
6. Gaining conscious control over the corset muscle (transverse abdominus) is the foundation of the ten exercises designed to strengthen your spine and core.
7. Honor your body while doing the ten exercises. If the exercise is mildly uncomfortable that is okay; however, if it is sharp then your body may not be strong enough to start exercising yet. Try it again in another week.

CHAPTER 6

Mental-Emotional Pain

In this chapter you likely are going to learn a completely new way of thinking about back pain. This is honestly the last thing I used to resolve the last of my back pain, and I really wish it was the first thing I did. I had some really significant mental-emotional resistance to healing, and with many things I had tried I just could not completely resolve the pain.

I also have seen this with many of my patients with chronic pain. Throughout my career as a therapist, I constantly was trying to understand why some people would just not get better, why their pain would not go away. They tried everything and had been to numerous doctors and still the pain would hold on. Some things they would do might have alleviated their pain somewhat but still the pain would hold on. It was this puzzle I just felt I *needed* to figure out.

At one point in my career, I had seen two patients, both of whom had had knee replacements and were around the same age. They had had their knees done within hours of each other with the same doctor and the same prosthetic. The one difference was they had vastly different healing experiences.

One patient was walking across the whole gym the first day and the other could barely take ten steps on the first day because the pain was so high. The first patient was discharged from therapy a full month and a half sooner than the second, and was completely pain free! Watching these vastly different healing experiences between these two patients left me unsettled. The memory rolled around in my brain for years as I tried to make sense of it. It took quite some time for me to understand this scenario. Eventually I pieced together some understanding of why different people can heal so differently. The foundation, or basis, I have found that causes this difference in healing is their mental-emotional state.

Fast-forward a few years and I learn about EFT or Emotional Freedom Technique. EFT originally was designed to eliminate phobias. When I initially had learned about EFT I was *very* skeptical. This was a crazy approach of banging away at specific points on the face and body that are supposed to correlate with certain meridian points.

My opinion changed drastically as I watched a colleague who was deathly afraid of bees lose this phobia in about ten minutes with EFT. My attention definitely was caught. I knew from experience, just the mention of a bee would send this woman screaming out of the room whether or not she actually had seen it. After this experience, I learned as much as I could about EFT and tried it on anything and everything. I mean, let's face it, your emotions play such an important role in your everyday life. If those emotions can be calmed down then your day is going to be more pleasant. I was determined to make my days more pleasant!

I started noticing many positive effects on my emotions with the use of EFT, and it did not take long before I started trying it on my physical pain. I was fully aware of how emotional an experience pain could be so I thought it would be worth a shot.

I did not notice an immediate difference in my physical aches and pains and I abandoned the idea of using EFT for my pain until my experience in Colorado. I had taken a travel assignment out to Colorado, and the first thing I had noticed in the area was the general mental-emotional attitude was somehow happier. After a week or so of working with the patients in the area I had patients coming back to me after one, two, maybe three sessions saying they were all better and they did not need to come back anymore.

I was absolutely flabbergasted. The first time it happened, I thought the patient was lying to me. I actually tried to talk them back into their pain. I asked questions such as, "Are you sure?", and even said, "That is not possible, it does not work way". I was so absolutely stunned because these same issues would take months to heal with the patients I see in Ohio. I did the exact same treatment plan with the Colorado patients as I did with the ones in Ohio. Patients getting better in two to three visits was a regular occurrence out there in Colorado, and I was completely puzzled as to how this was occurring.

I initially attributed these amazing results to the fact these people were more active in general than the people in Ohio; which, on the whole, was true. However, I did not think that was the whole reason because I did work with some quite active people in Ohio and they did not get these same results. The only thing markedly different was the mental-emotional attitude of the two groups.

This area was notably healthier and more well-adjusted mentally and emotionally and I was not the only person to notice this. A physician I was working with actually moved his family out there from New England because he wanted them to grow up in a healthier mental environment. I concluded there was a strong connection between our mental-emotional attitude and our ability to heal.

This experience had re-awakened my desire to get EFT to work for the physical body; more specifically, *my* physical body. With some determination, I started using EFT once again to get rid of my own physical problems. I slowly started noticing some changes in my back pain. It took me some time to really figure out the tricks for incorporating EFT into healing back pain but I eventually did. Now you are going to enjoy the fruits of my labor and learn how to use this technique successfully. You also will learn about the pitfalls that can get in your way and decrease EFT's effectiveness.

First, you are going to learn how to do EFT. Then I will guide you through the process to use it on your chronic back pain. EFT is performed by gently tapping on specific meridian points of the body. The meridian system is basically a roadmap of the body's energy pathways. Somehow, tapping on specific points helps stimulate these energy pathways, which can have profound effects on the body itself; however, the effects are subtle. Now, when I say gentle tapping that is exactly what I mean. There is no need to damage or hurt yourself during this process.

A round of EFT begins with the set up procedure. It is necessary to prepare your energetic system and dissolve any resistance. To do the set up procedure you tap on a point on the inside of the hand just above the pinky finger, which is called the Karate Chop Point.

To visualize it, imagine someone doing a karate chop. The part of the hand they hit with is where the Karate Chop Point is located. While gently tapping on this point at the side of the hand you repeat some of the following phrases addressing your pain. Use the phrase or phrases that feel the most comfortable to you. If you feel uncomfortable with the phrase then the positive effects can be minimized, so it is important you use the phrase most comfortable to you.

"Even though I am experiencing back pain, I deeply love and accept myself anyway."
"Even though I am feeling back pain, I am open to accepting myself anyway."
"Even though I have experienced back pain, I am open to loving and accepting myself *now*."

You can change out the phrase back pain for a description that may fit you better. Some examples people have used include: stabbing pain in my back, shooting pain in my leg, a screwdriver is driving in my back, this deep ache in my butt and back, a throbbing back, pain like a toothache, tightness in my back, my back locks up, my back muscles feel tired, etc. I am sure you can come up with one that really fits you and your experience.

As you choose a phrase that suits you, use one that really describes the feeling so you can allow yourself to really feel the emotions associated with the pain you are experiencing. It is these emotions you are going to release, so you really have to bring them to the front of your mind. Then the magic can happen and the emotional charge goes away.

Whichever setup phrase you choose, repeat that phrase three to five times before you tap through the remaining points with the phrase you have chosen. In my case, the phrase is "back pain." In your case it can be anything, ranging from as simple as "back pain" to as detailed as "a screwdriver is driving in my back."

The remaining thirteen points are as follows. If you want to see pictures of the different points then you can refer to the picture index at the back of the book. It is always nice to have a good visual to understand what you are doing. So do not hesitate to flip to the picture index.

EB = beginning of the eyebrow, which I refer to as inside of the eye
SE = side of the eye, which I refer to as outside of the eye
UE = under the eye
UN = under the nose
Ch = chin
CB = beginning of the collarbone
UA = under the arm
BN = below the nipple
Th = thumb
IF = index finger
MF = middle finger
BF = baby finger
KC = karate chop point

Using all thirteen points is the original way EFT was designed by founder Gary Craig.. To save time I shortened the round and eliminated all the hand points (Th, IF, MF and BF). I just tap both wrists together instead. I find using just nine points streamlines the process; however, if it feels better for you to use all of the points then feel free.

In addition, I have removed the BN point below the nipple point from my general protocol. I have found the location caused some embarrassment with some of the more sensitive clients. Since it is important to feel as comfortable as possible while doing EFT, the easiest solution was to just eliminate the BN point. However, if you really want to keep that point as part of your overall protocol then please feel free to do so. It is a good meridian to address since it is related to the liver and to anger in general.

So, as an example, I am going to take you through a session of back pain tapping:

Tapping on the Karate Chop Point I want you to repeat:

"Even though I have this stabbing sharp pain in my back I am open to accepting myself anyway."

"Even though I have this stabbing sharp pain in my back I am open to accepting myself anyway."

"Even though I have this stabbing sharp pain in my back I love and accept myself deeply and completely."

Tap at the inside of the eye, saying, "This sharp and stabbing pain in my back."

Really allow yourself to feel the pain in your back and how it affects your emotions.

Tap at the outside of the eye, saying, "This sharp and stabbing pain in my back."

Tap beneath the eye, saying, "This sharp and stabbing pain in my back."

Tap beneath the nose, saying, "This sharp and stabbing pain in my back."

Tap at the chin, saying, "This sharp and stabbing pain in my back."

Tap at the collarbone, saying, "This sharp and stabbing pain in my back."

Tap under the arm, saying, "This sharp and stabbing pain in my back."

Tap the wrists together, saying, "This sharp and stabbing pain in my back."

Tap the Karate Chop Point, saying, "This sharp and stabbing pain in my back."

Then take some three to five deep breaths and you can incorporate the sigh-like breath for this.

After a few repetitions of this you will notice your pain is less intense and less stabbing. It may change in quality, maybe to more of an ache than a stab. At this point you can go through the procedure again with your special description–ache, throb, nagging, etc. This should give you a great foundation for using EFT to manage your back pain. The EFT technique can be taken much further; however, you need to get comfortable with the basics. Essentially, you have to walk before you can run.

One thing I want to emphasize during this process is you really want to connect with the feeling–the emotions associated with the pain you are feeling. This is one of the biggest pitfalls people experience with EFT, myself included. They try staying emotionally detached from the experience. Of course it makes sense, because when you are in pain for long periods of time you learn how to tune it out. Now you have to tune it in so you can eliminate it. No worries because you will not have to tune in very long before the quality of the pain changes with the tapping.

LEARNING POINTS CHAPTER 6

1. Your mental-emotional state can drastically affect your ability to heal quickly and effectively.
2. Emotional Freedom Technique (EFT) can be used to address the mental-emotional side of your pain.
3. EFT consists of a set-up at the Karate Chop Point and thirteen tapping points, or my abbreviated nine points.
4. It is important for best results to "tune into" your emotional pain while tapping for your physical pain. This can be difficult to do because chronic pain sufferers such as yourself tend to "tune out" as much pain as possible.

CHAPTER 7

Help Me Heal

I totally agree with you, this healing process is a J-O-B. It is not a picnic. Look at how much you have learned so far, which really is a lot. You have learned about your back's anatomy and the sacroiliac joint, why the sacroiliac joint is important, how to address your muscle spasms, how to retrain the sacroiliac joint, developing good muscular support and addressing the mental-emotional aspects of back pain. You should congratulate yourself. You definitely have come a long way and you definitely should see some results by now.

We are almost ready to wrap it up; however, one more thing will really allow this healing process to go as smoothly as possible. This final thing is having someone put their hands on you and do some bodywork to help your healing process along. The strengthening process can be uncomfortable. Depending on how long it has been since the muscles have worked properly, they may be working themselves into quite a tizzy trying to get stronger and keep up with all the big boy muscles. Having someone help you through this process can speed it along and make the whole process much more comfortable.

A bodyworker is anyone who actively uses their hands to make changes with someone's body, also considered manipulative therapy. Using the term "bodyworker" keeps it separate from a massage therapist, even though a massage therapist is considered a bodyworker. When most people think of a massage therapist they immediately think of a relaxation massage, which is not the intention here. A relaxation massage has its place; however, it is not exactly what you are looking for in this healing process. You want a bodyworker who will help you make the muscle, joint and postural changes necessary for your healing.

The process of finding the right bodyworker can be intimidating, so you are going to be given all the information you need to find the best one for your needs. You are going to become familiar with the different disciplines or practitioners who do bodywork, the most common forms of bodywork techniques, and how to choose the best practitioner or technique for your needs.

A variety of disciplines or practitioners can do the bodywork you need to heal. These disciplines are as follows:
Massage Therapist
Physical Therapist (also called physiotherapists)
Occupational Therapist
Chiropractor
Osteopath

Some of the popular bodywork techniques include:

Craniosacral Therapy
Myofascial Release
Active Release Techniques®
Visceral Manipulation
Trigger Point Therapy
Chiropractic Adjustments
Reiki

And some I am not as familiar with:

Rolfing®

Alexander Technique®
Bioenergetics
Bowen Technique®
Feldenkrais®
Hakomi®
Postural Integration
Shiatsu
Structural Integration
Somatic Experiencing®
Trager® Approach
Polarity Therapy
Rebalancing

Throughout the following section you will get a description of these popular bodywork techniques to help you decide what is most appropriate for you. Keep in mind as your body changes and heals, you may need different bodywork techniques, or you may not need any at all. Let's go through each technique, starting with Craniosacral Therapy.

Craniosacral Therapy strongly impacts the nervous system, specifically between the cranium (the head) and the sacrum (triangle bone at the pelvis). Historically, there has been significant controversy whether the bones in the head are able to move.

Originally, physicians were taught the bones in the head only moved in young infants and fused solidly in adults. Research performed in the 1970s by Dr. John Upledger, D.O. found there indeed is space between the cranial bones and very subtle movement occurs. It also was discovered the whole nervous system from head to tail has a subtle rhythmic movement.

Craniosacral Therapy uses a *very* gentle touch, only five grams of pressure, which is about the weight of a quarter. The effects of Craniosacral Therapy can vary somewhat since you are dealing with the nervous system, which can add an element of unpredictability. The technique itself is instrumental in re-establishing the rhythm of the central nervous system between the head (cranium) and the triangle bone (sacrum). The rhythm can get skewed when there is prolonged back pain and injury, such as what you are experiencing.

Craniosacral Therapy also allows the nervous system to re-organize itself, which stimulates the body's ability to heal. Craniosacral Therapy is commonly performed by physical therapists and massage therapists; however it also is performed by occupational therapists, nurses, osteopaths and chiropractors.

How do you know if Craniosacral Therapy is right for you? I will share with you the indicators I use for applying this technique before the others.

One is if you are too sore to tolerate much pressure and the thought of being touched makes you nervous.
Another is if your pain is diffuse and not specifically located in any one spot. This technique affects a broad area, so if you are aching all over then this may be the best one for you to start with.

To find a bodyworker skilled in Craniosacral Therapy go to the website www.upledger.com and click on "find a therapist." That will take you to a page where you click on "find a practitioner" and from that page you can do a search. On the right, under "search by modality," select "Craniosacral Therapy / SomatoEmotional Release" and on the left, put your state or zip code. This should allow you to find a local provider.

Keep in mind, even if you cannot find a local bodyworker listed in the directory, you always can try calling local physical therapist and massage therapy clinics and ask if they have specialists. Many times it is quite costly to be a part of directories so many bodyworkers choose not to participate.

Next, we are going to cover the technique called Myofascial Release. This technique targets the body's fascial system. Yes, I did say fascia. It is pronounced "faaasha". Let me give you a visual of the fascia. When you are looking at a steak it is the silvery stuff between the different cuts of the meat. It can be the stringy and tough part of the meat. The fascia creates a three-dimensional web going from the tip of the toes to the tip of the head. It surrounds each and every organ, muscle, bone, nerve and blood vessel.

The fascia has a lot of elasticity to it, allowing movement between all the different structures. However, through injury, inflammation and poor posture the fascia can get solidified and shortened and lose its elasticity. This is essentially scar tissue, which can place up to two thousand pounds of pressure on any structure such as a nerve, artery or muscle. That really is a lot of pressure. I am certain you can see how two thousand pounds of pressure around sensitive structures such as nerves and arteries can practically strangle them to death, causing them to do all sorts of crazy things–go numb, cause pain, etc.

Muscles may not be highly sensitive; however, if they have to work against two thousand pounds of pressure that is a lot of work. They will get exhausted much more quickly than they should. That is when you feel tiredness in the muscles even though it seems like you did very little. Once there is scar tissue in the fascia it affects other areas of the body, much like a snag in a sweater can affect a part of the sweater far away from the original snag.

You know how you can get a snag in the bottom of a sweater and the threads all the way up in the shoulder area are affected? It is the same way with the fascia. This can stress a number of areas of the body as well, and make it even harder and more tiring to move. For example, you may notice you have the original injury on the right side of your lower back. Now you notice discomfort going down your right leg and up the right side of your ribcage. Your right arm may tire out quickly without much exertion. This is likely the strain caused from the original injury in the fascia on the right side of the lower back.

Now that you have a basic understanding of the fascia you easily can figure out Myofascial Release is for releasing the fascia. It targets those restrictions and scar tissue that cause the two thousand pounds of pressure in the fascia. While you are receiving Myofascial Release the touch is much firmer than Craniosacral Therapy. You will feel a lot of pulling; however, it is not overly forceful and usually not painful or only mildly painful.

Myofascial Release is commonly performed by physical therapists, since the technique originally was designed by a physical therapist. However, it also is performed by occupational therapists, massage therapists and, less commonly, by nurses, osteopaths and chiropractors.

How do you know if Myofascial Release is right for you? I will share with you the indicators I use for approaching someone with this technique before the others:

One is if the pain from the injury spans a larger area of the body but not throughout the whole body.

Another is if the pain goes in a criss-cross pattern from the front of the body to the back and from left to right. This criss-cross pattern clearly indicates Myofascial Release may be appropriate to use.

Another is if the area to be treated is not hypersensitive and can tolerate moderate and firm pressure. The pain has been there for a long time and the longer it has been present that pain has shown up in other areas of the body (like pulling a snag on a sweater).

There are two ways to find a Myofascial Release Bodyworker.

The first way is as follows:
Go to the website www.upledger.com and click on "find a therapist." That will take you to a page where you click on "find a practitioner" and from that page you can do a search. On the right under "search by modality," select "Myofascial Release" and on the left put your state or zip code. This should allow you to find a local provider.

The second way is a little bit easier:
Go to the website www.mfrtherapist.com and from there you can search by state.

Keep in mind, even if you cannot find a local bodyworker listed in the directory you always can try calling local physical therapist and massage therapy clinics and ask if they have specialists. Many times it is quite costly to be a part of these directories so many bodyworkers choose not to participate.

Now let's discuss ActiveRelease Techniques®, which is a form of Myofascial Release. The major difference between ActiveRelease Techniques® and standard Myofascial Release is ActiveRelease is extremely specific. If there is scar tissue, or a tight muscle, tendon, nerve or ligament, ActiveRelease can break up that restriction quickly and restore normal movement to that specific area. It is common that the scar tissue will cause a nerve to stick to something it is not supposed to, such as a muscle, bone or tendon. ActiveRelease effectively can break up this scar tissue so normal movement can be restored. Then once again the nerves, muscles, tendons, etc. are happy and able to do their jobs without getting pulled back from the scar tissue and other nearby muscles.

ActiveRelease Techniques® is a highly effective technique that works quickly once the scar tissue is located. Compared to the Craniosacral and Myofascial Release the touch is deep and can be aggressive. It can be simply amazing just how quickly the results are felt by the client and how movement can be restored within minutes.

For many other techniques it could take several sessions to get such results. The major drawback is ActiveRelease Techniques® can be quite painful. It is almost as though you are concentrating the pain from five sessions all into one. The pain is better almost immediately after ActiveRelease is completed; however, the pain itself can be a limiting factor during treatment. In addition, since the technique is so specific in the areas it affects, I have found many times a broader technique such as Craniosacral or Myofascial Release is good to do prior to ActiveRelease to increase its effectiveness.

ActiveRelease Techniques® requires specific certification. The majority of providers are certified chiropractors since the technique originally was designed by a chiropractor. However, massage therapists, physical therapists, occupational therapists, osteopaths, and even nurses can perform ActiveRelease.

How do you know if ActiveRelease Techniques® is right for you? I will share with you the indicators I use for utilizing this technique first and foremost before others.

One is if the painful area is small and localized.

Another is if you do not have much time and want to get as much as possible done in a short period of time.

Another is if you are willing and able to tolerate higher amounts of pain to reach your goals.

To find an ActiveRelease Techniques® provider near you, check out the website www.activerelease.com. You will see a tab saying "find a provider." Then you will see a tab called "ART providers by location" where you can find a local provider by using your zip code.

The next technique you get to learn about is Visceral Manipulation. I know it is a mouthful and, thankfully, it is easier to explain than it is to say. Basically, the viscera is the organs of the body, such as the lungs, heart, intestines, bladder, stomach, etc. Visceral Manipulation is a technique specialized to address specifically the organs inside your abdomen. Each organ has normal movement in which it participates. If the movement is impaired, that can result in pain and oftentimes severe difficulties in standing or sitting up straight.

The abdominal area is quite close to the lower back, especially the lower organs of the intestines, kidneys and bladder. So these organs can be affected by injury to the lower back. Visceral Manipulation commonly is performed by osteopaths, since the technique originally was designed by an osteopathic physician; however, it also is performed by physical therapists, occupational therapists, massage therapists and, less commonly, by nurses or chiropractors.

How do you know if Visceral Manipulation is right for you? I will share with you the indicators I use for approaching someone with this technique first and foremost before the others.

One is if significant pain is located in the abdomen area.
Another is if you have difficulty sitting up or standing straight, feeling as though there is too much tightness in the front of the body holding you hunched over.

Another is if feel pressure in your back and cannot pinpoint it to any specific location or muscle area.

To find a bodyworker skilled in Visceral Manipulation go to the website www.upledger.com and on click on the tab saying "find a therapist." That will take you to a page where you click on "find a practitioner" and from that page you can do a search. On the right, under "search by modality," select "Visceral Manipulation" and on the left, put your state or zip code. This should allow you to find a local provider.

Keep in mind, even if you cannot find a local bodyworker listed in the directory you always can try calling local physical therapist and massage therapy clinics and asking if they have specialists. Many times it is quite costly to be a part of these directories and there are many bodyworkers choose not to participate so it is not a waste of time to try calling local providers.

A few more techniques are left to cover and the next one is Trigger Point Therapy. Trigger Point Therapy specifically addresses the muscles and does not address ligaments, nerves, tendons or fascia.

The basic idea with this technique is placing direct pressure on a muscle that is tight or spastic will cause it to relax. I know this sounds completely backwards, but it works. I have been doing it for close to twenty years with people and I have had it done to myself as well. The spasms commonly are caused from muscles being overworked. As the body is healing, it is easy for a muscle to get overworked. After a few moments, you will completely understand why this happens.

Muscles are very specific in how they strengthen. If muscles are always in one position, then they will strengthen in that position specifically. I want you to recall earlier when we did that retraining move for the pelvis (sacroiliac joint). Following retraining of the pelvis, numerous muscles are moving differently because of this new positioning. These same muscles are strong and competent in the position that had been painful and dysfunctional; however, once placed in a different position the muscles no longer have that same strength. These same muscles now need to be re-strengthened.

So now these weaker muscles have to run to catch up to the stronger muscles around them. They get themselves all worked up into a tizzy and end up being tight and spastic. Unfortunately, when muscles are stuck in a spasm they are not able to strengthen effectively, so it is best to break that tight spastic cycle. A great way to break free from the tight spastic cycle is using Trigger Point Therapy.

A great benefit to this technique is it is widely practiced, especially among massage therapists. Trigger Point Therapy is usually part of the standard training in massage therapy school. In addition to massage therapists many other disciplines also commonly perform Trigger Point Therapy, including physical therapists, occupational therapists, chiropractors and nurses.

How do you know if Trigger Point Therapy is right for you? I will share with you the indicators I use for approaching someone with this technique first and foremost before the others.

The first is if the tightness is localized deep in the muscles around the pelvic and back area; especially in the buttocks.

Another is if the tightness and discomfort tends to feel better in the morning and get worse as the day wears on or with vigorous activity.

Another is if stretching feels good and then it seems the muscles tighten right back up.

The best way to find someone skilled in Trigger Point Therapy would be contacting your local massage therapists. Ask if they are familiar with the technique and, if so, how long they have been doing it. It is best to find someone who has done it for at least a few years. It is also beneficial to use tools to manage your trigger points on a daily basis, which will allow for faster healing. You will learn all about using tools to manage your trigger points in the next chapter.

Now let's talk about Chiropractic Adjustments. I am not a chiropractor so I will not go into a tremendous amount of detail here; however, adjustments of the spine can play an important role in the healing process. As you get the pelvis, which is like the foundation of a house, leveled out and working properly again, the joints stacked above the pelvis (the spine) may need some help in getting lined up properly. In addition, the tailbone also can get out of whack with chronic back pain and many chiropractors can address a problem with the tailbone. Similar adjustments also can be done by osteopaths and some physical therapists.

How do you know if a Chiropractic Adjustments are right for you? I will share with you some indicators I use to refer a client to a chiropractor for an adjustment.

The first is if there is a "catch" in the spine with specific movements.

Another is if there is pain right on the tailbone area and if you touch it you can tell it is shifted to one side.

Another is if there are restrictions in your ability to turn your spine from side to side.

It is not difficult to find a local chiropractor who can give you a good adjustment; however, if you find you are not comfortable with someone after the first adjustment, maybe you need to find another chiropractor. There is nothing wrong with finding a chiropractor, or any health care provider for matter, who is a good and comfortable fit for you.

Reiki is the next form of bodywork. It is done primarily with a hands-off approach. Reiki works primarily with the body's energy systems and is a very subtle and gentle approach to relieving pain. Reiki also can relax the body, which helps to turn on the body's self-healing mechanisms. Reiki can be done while doing another form of massage or bodywork listed above. In those cases, it does increase the effectiveness of the technique tremendously. Reiki does not require any specific licensing; however, it does have a certification program with three levels of strength and expertise. It commonly is practiced by massage therapists since it complements the massages wonderfully.

How do you know if Reiki is right for you? I will share with you some indicators I use to choose Reiki as my primary form of treatment.

The first is if you are highly sensitive to touch and would rather have a hands-off approach.

Another is if you are very nervous and agitated and primarily need stress relief to allow the healing process to begin or continue.

Another is if you have a fear of being touched and still want treatment.

The easiest way to find a Reiki practitioner would be contacting your local massage therapist. Ask him or her if they are certified to do Reiki or if they know of someone who is certified.

I know it can be a bit daunting to find the right bodyworker for you. The information you have received will make the process much easier. Knowing what you need is the first step in finding who you need to help you. :-)

LEARNING POINTS FOR CHAPTER SEVEN

1. A bodyworker can help make your healing process more comfortable.
2. A bodyworker is anyone who uses their hands to make changes to someone's body, also considered manipulative therapy.
3. A variety of disciplines or practitioners can do the bodywork you need to heal. These disciplines are as follows: Massage Therapist, Physical Therapist (also called Physiotherapist), Occupational Therapist, Chiropractor and Osteopath.
4. Some of the popular bodywork techniques used include: Craniosacral Therapy, Myofascial Release, ActiveRelease Techniques®, Visceral Mobilization, Trigger Point Release, Chiropractic Adjustments and Reiki.
5. Knowing what you need is the first step in finding who you need to help you.

Chapter 8

Tools for Trigger Points

Trigger points are a normal occurrence during the healing process. As muscles adjust to new movement patterns, they tend to develop trigger points, which are basically tight spastic muscles that are fairly specific in their locations. These are nothing to be worried about because, as the muscles adjust and strengthen to the new patterns, the trigger points will resolve themselves; however, until process is completed it can be quite uncomfortable. In this regard, it is of great benefit if you can alleviate your trigger points regularly on your own. Specific trigger point tools can be used daily to release your tight, spastic muscles.

I know it is amazing to have someone alleviate these trigger points for you and that really cannot be replaced. However, it may difficult to find the time or the money to go to someone daily throughout your healing process. Instead, you can use trigger point tools on your own for daily relief.

Before using any Trigger Point tools, many have found receiving at least one treatment from a professional trained in Trigger Point Therapy is very helpful in understanding how to use the correct pressure for the best result. You also can get an idea of what to expect as your muscles let go from the spastic tightness once the trigger points are released. Refer to the previous chapter to learn how to find a Trigger Point Therapy practitioner for you.

A variety of tools available for self-management of trigger points. You are going to learn about some of the most popular tools, which happen to be my favorites. The three tools you are going to learn about are the Theracane, the Jacknobber and the Miracle Balls. All three have different benefits and uses and you will learn which one may be best for your needs.

One of the most popular tools is the Theracane. It is designed in a hook shape so you have the leverage you need to release Trigger Points in the backside of your body. This tool is great for getting those hard to reach spots you cannot touch with your hands.

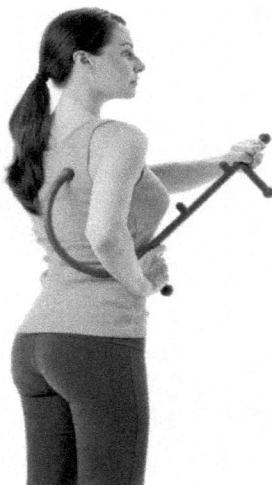

Another favorite of mine is the Jacknobber, which is shaped like a jack. It allows you to get a comfortable grip as you use it on different muscles in your body. This tool is great to use so your hand does not get fatigued while releasing Trigger Points in the areas you can reach.

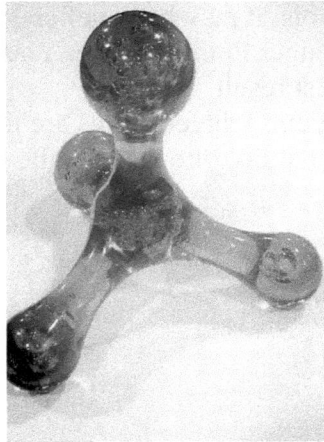

However, an absolute favorite of mine is the Miracle Ball Method by Elaine Petrone, which consists of two vinyl balls and a small manual. These balls are just the right size to get into the hip muscles and the lower back. I like them the best because you can relax your body and roll around to find Trigger Points in your lower back and hip areas. I have seen the Miracle Ball Method at Amazon.com, Walmart and Target so they are very accessible. If you would prefer to use a household item, tennis balls have worked for many people. Personally, I find them to be a bit too small and too hard to really work for me; however, many people have reported successfully releasing their Trigger Points with them. If you happen to have a tennis ball handy, then it will not hurt to try using it to release you own Trigger Points.

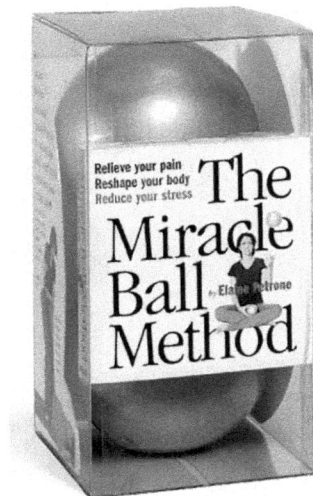

LEARNING POINTS FOR CHAPTER 8

1. As muscles adjust to new movement patterns, they tend to develop Trigger Points.

2. Trigger Points are basically tight, spastic muscles that are fairly specific in their locations.

3. Trigger Points can be uncomfortable and it would be beneficial for you to use tools daily to get rid of them.

4. Before using any Trigger Point tools, it may be beneficial for you to have at least one treatment with a professional trained in Trigger Point Release. You will gain increased insight into what kind of pressure to use for the best result.

5. Three effective tools to alleviate your Trigger Points are the Theracane, the Jacknobber and the Miracle Balls Method. My personal favorite is using the Miracle Balls.

Chapter 9

Wrapping It Up

The techniques I have discussed with you are far from being exhaustive of everything available. They are the techniques I have found the most beneficial and helpful with myself and my clients. That in no way negates the effectiveness of techniques I have not personally experienced. If you happen to know of a technique that is spectacularly effective for you, then please do not hesitate to use it. However, if you are seeking out something different, I would highly recommend any of the aforementioned techniques. I know from experience they do indeed work and help in the healing process for back pain.

So, in the all-inclusive, seven-step system you learned how to get rid of your muscle spasms using a few tricks, including magnesium, breathing techniques and natural or pharmaceutical anti-inflammatories. You also learned the retraining technique I have used on my clients for almost ten years now with amazing results. The retraining includes using a supportive sacroiliac belt as needed.

Numerous exercises help support all these changes at the sacroiliac joint and each exercise is a necessary part of the healing process. The process does not stop with the exercises because if you do not address the mental-emotional aspects of your pain you could be blocking your own healing. Using EFT (Emotional Freedom Technique) will help address the healing of the mental-emotional aspects. If you still need a bit of help in the healing process, using a bodyworker to help you may be a brilliant choice. In chapter seven you were given all the tools you need to find the right bodyworker to help with relaxing your muscles and facilitating healing.

If you are having difficulty putting this all together and have questions, then you can contact me at lisa@lisamariekeller.com and we can set up a time for consult.

I want to emphasis to you that the healing process does take time. For the number of years you have had chronic pain it likely will take that number of months to resolve your pain. Another point I did not bring up earlier is there may be some fatigue involved with the healing process. This is different from normal everyday fatigue, and may be accompanied by a bit of a brain fog–like it is just difficult to think. You really will crave sleep during this time. That is normal, okay, and even desirable.

Your body does its best healing while sleeping, so it is normal and natural for the body to crave sleep while it is healing. You may want to set aside a little extra time to sleep during this time to facilitate the healing process a bit more. I know this can be difficult because it was for me. However, the benefits outweigh the inconveniences. The rest will be most welcomed by your body.

Thank you for taking the time to heal yourself from back pain. I would love to hear from you and the results you have received. Do not hesitate to email me at lisa@lisamariekeller.com or you can post comments on the Facebook page:

https://www.facebook.com/LisaMarieKellerDesignYourHealth

I do regularly check the Facebook page and I will respond to your comments when I am able. I love hearing how the seven steps have affected your life and your back pain so please let me know!

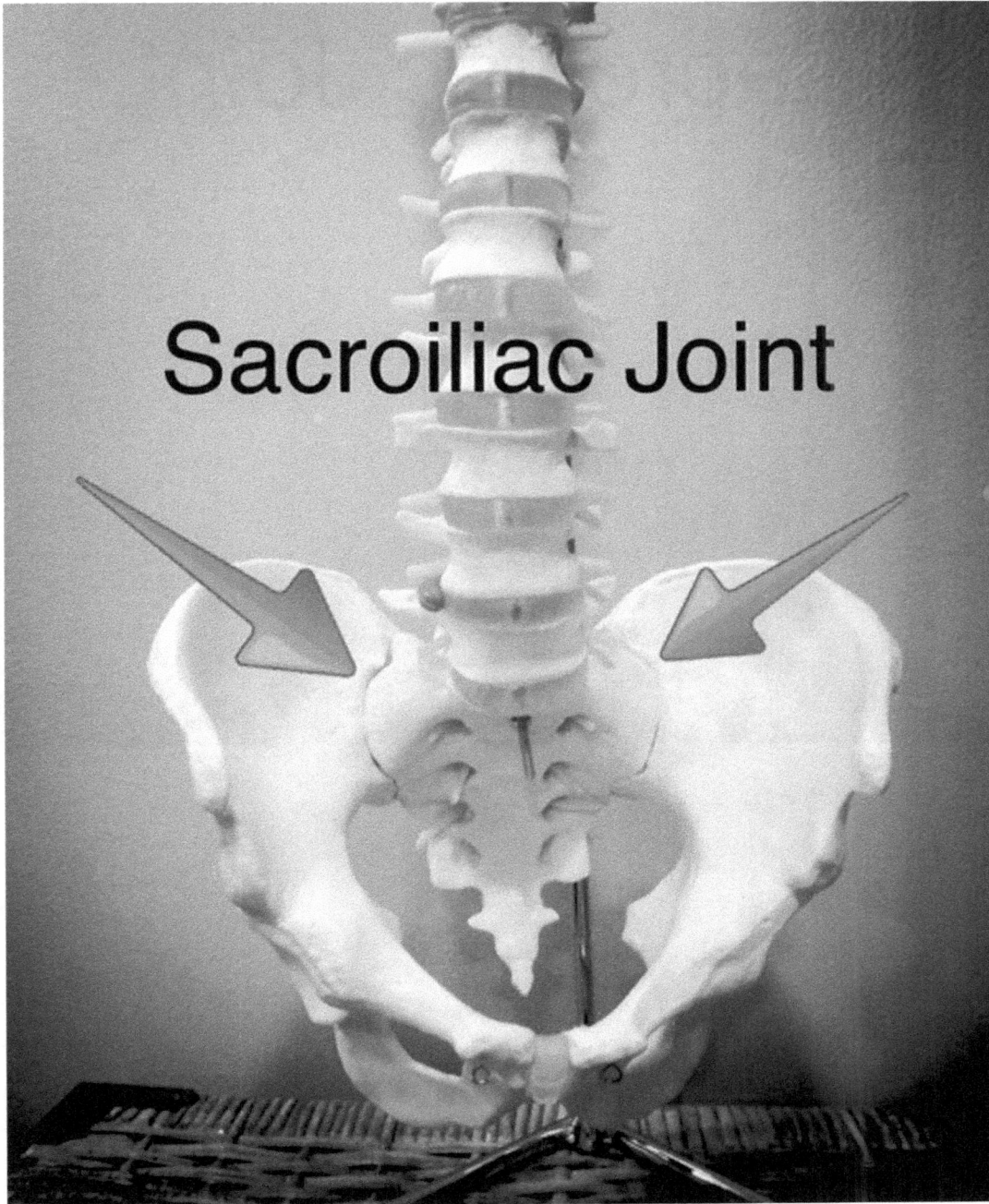

Sacroiliac Joint

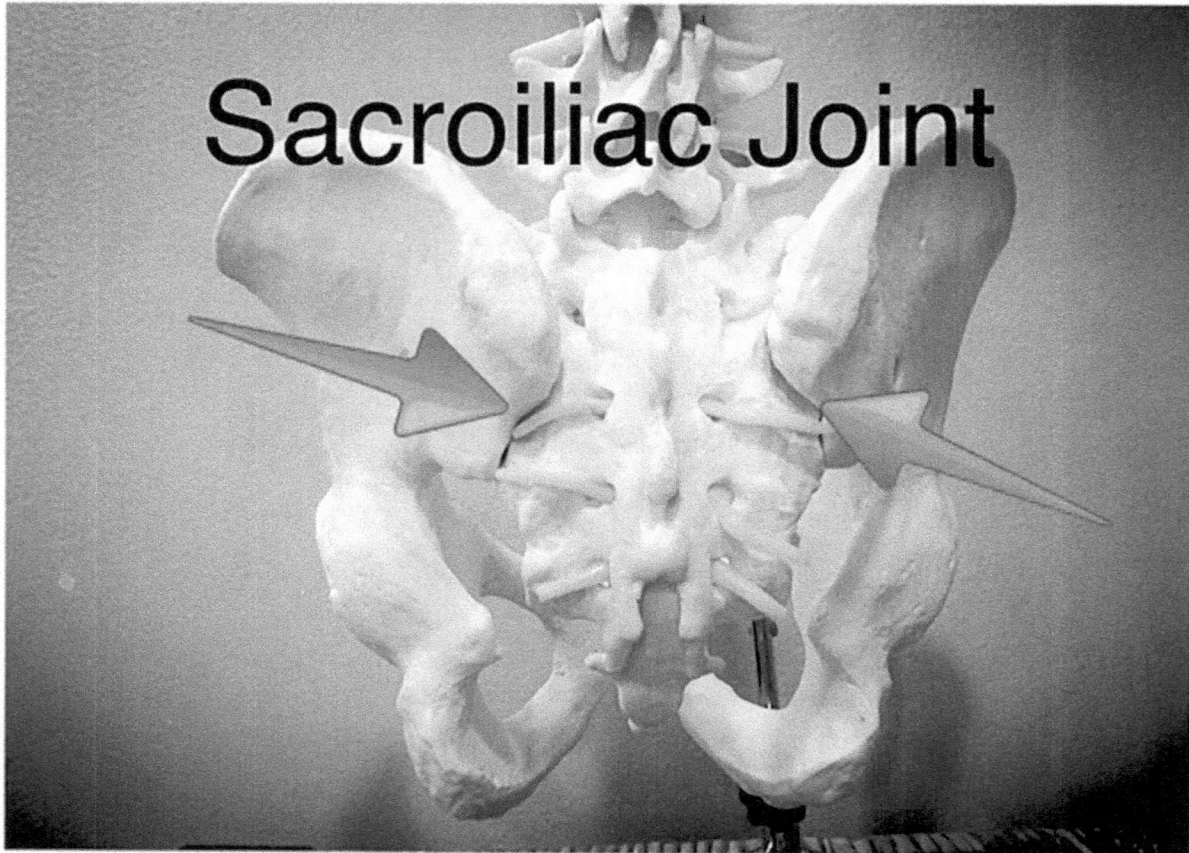

Sacroiliac Joint

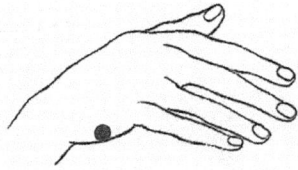

The KC Point

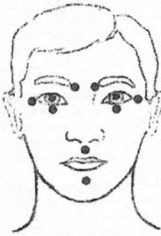

ED, SE, UE, UN and CH Points

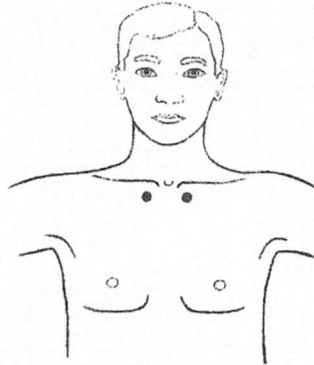

The CB Points

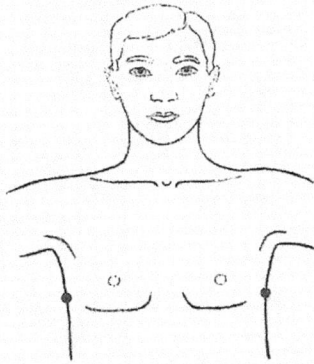

The UA Points

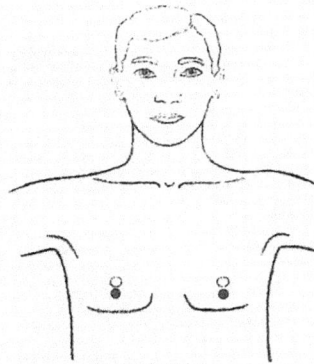

The BN Points

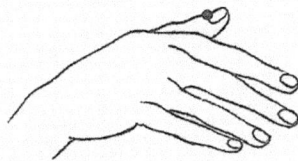

The Th Point

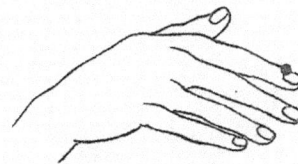

The IF Point

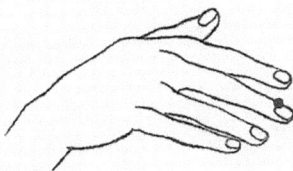

The MF Point

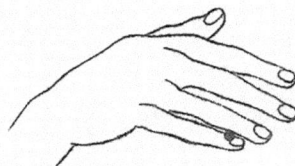

The BF Point

www.ingramcontent.com/pod-product-compliance
Lightning Source LLC
Chambersburg PA
CBHW080621270326
41928CB00016B/3148